Handbook of
Clinical Methods
in Communication Disorders

Handbook of Clinical Methods in Communication Disorders

William R. Leith, PhD
Wayne State University

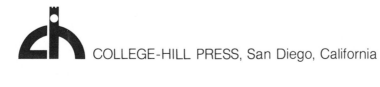

COLLEGE-HILL PRESS, San Diego, California

College-Hill Press
4284 41st Street
San Diego, California 92105

Library of Congress Cataloging in Publication Data

Leith, William
    Handbook of clinical methods in communication disorders.

    Bibliography: p.
    Includes index.
    1. Speech Therapy. 2. Therapist and patient. 3. Communicative disorders—Treatment. I. Title. [DNLM: 1. Language disorders—Therapy—Handbooks.
2. Speech disorders—Therapy—Handbooks. 3. Language therapy—Handbooks.
4. Speech therapy—Handbooks. WM
475 L533h]
RC423.L414   1983   616.85'506   83-23134

ISBN 0-933014-91-0

Printed in the United States of America

*This book is dedicated to
all of my clients
who taught me how to do therapy
and to
all of my students
who taught me how to share this information.*

Preface

As a speech clinician university professor with over 30 years of experience, I have been concerned for many years with the effectiveness, or sometimes the lack thereof, of our professional services. My concern has not been with our academic information, but, rather, with our lack of clinical information.

Our profession has made great strides during the 50 years it has been in existence. We have researched deeply into the etiologies of the various disorders; we have devised numerous diagnostic instruments; we have advanced into the area of language disorders; we have studied carefully the speech and language process. However, there seems to be one crucial facet of our profession that has escaped our attention. That is the therapeutic process itself. We have been so preoccupied with the study of the disorders themselves that we have paid scant attention to the process through which the disorders are remediated. From our research and empirical base, we know what new speech behaviors to introduce to our clients; but the *how* of therapy remains a mystical procedure. We learn it through observations of other clinicians and through experiences in the clinic room. To say the least, it is not a well understood process. Perhaps, because of the vagueness of the process, we have very little insight into the most frustrating of all clinical problems; that is, the difficulty in achieving carry-over of new speech behaviors into the client's natural speaking environments.

The history of any profession functions primarily to familiarize members of that profession with past accomplishments and failures. Having this information, future generations of the profession can embark from this point of professional development, and not repeat all of the trials and errors their predecessors made. As I attempted to share my clinical history with my students so that they would not repeat my clinical trials and errors, I discovered that I had neither the vocabulary nor the clinical concepts necessary for this sharing. I found myself limited to sharing anecdotal clinical experiences, hoping that the students would learn, at least by rote memory, how to deal with specific clinical situations.

As I became more frustrated with this problem, I began to study therapeutic procedures carefully in an attempt to find a vehicle through which I could share my clinical history. I found answers in various principles of learning. By combining principles, I developed a theoretic framework that I refer to as the *Clinical Interaction Model*. This theoretical framework provides both the vocabulary and the concepts that allow me to share my clinical history with my students. I can explain, according to specific principles, what has transpired in a clinical interaction. The Clinical Interaction Model is the focus of this book.

This book is about therapy; not *what* new speech behaviors are to be introduced to the various types of clients that we work with, but rather, *how* these new speech behaviors are taught. We are not considering a *new* therapy approach. We are discussing the same therapy that good clinicians have been doing for years. However, the Clinical Interaction Model is a way to view therapy so that the clinical interaction can be understood as a predictable teaching/learning exchange between the clinician and the client.

Therapy is not a mystical procedure. It is a learning situation that is based on learning principles and these govern the interaction between the clinician and the client. Once these principles are understood, therapeutic interaction becomes a lawful process which can be planned and the outcome predicted. *This is main purpose of this book*: to set forth those principles which govern our clinical interactions. This information should provide the clinician not only with the necessary means of planning a logical treatment program, but also the insight necessary to solve procedural problems if a treatment program is not yielding the desired results.

It is my sincerest wish that the information included in this book is of value to you, the reader. My students and I have found that a more complete understanding of the Clinical Interaction Model increases the efficiency and the effectiveness of our therapy. The core of our profession is the practicing clinician, providing clinical services to those who have communication disorders. Our professional reputation rests directly on the efficiency and effectiveness of these services. I hope that the information I have shared with you has a positive influence on your clinical services.

William R. Leith

Acknowledgments

A book of this nature is dependent on the input of many people and I would like to thank them for their assistance. I first of all thank Dr. Mary Jane Dettman who guided me on the original idea for the book and consulted with me during the years of development of the book. I also want to thank all of my students in my course in Clinical Behavior Management at Wayne State University for their help in the further development of the concepts, diagrams, and the model in the book.

I could not have organized the materials without the professional consulting provided by Dr. Mae Taylor, Specialist in Communication Disorders, Utah State Office of Education, Salt Lake City, Utah; Mrs. Sue Laskowski, speech–language clinician in the schools in Utica, Michigan; Mrs. Denise Dinan, speech-language clinician in the schools in St. Clair Shores, Michigan; Miss Karen Schmanski, speech-language clinician in Bon Secours Hospital, Grosse Pointe, Michigan; and Mrs. Kristine Sbaschnig, Clinical Coordinator, Communication Disorders and Sciences, Wayne State University, Detroit, Michigan.

I would like to give special thanks to my class in Clinical Behavior Management at Wayne State University in the fall of 1982. They read the manuscript and provided invaluable editing. Teri Rutkowski worked with me on both editing and indexing for which I am very grateful.

Finally, I want to thank CVR for teaching me the importance of the clinician and therapy in my chosen profession.

Contents

SECTION II: THE "HOW" OF THERAPY

List of Figures

THE ESSENCE
OF THERAPY

Chapter 1

Synopsis

Compared to other professions, ours is still in its infancy. As with young children, we often ask, "Where did we come from?" We also sometimes question exactly what we do and how we do it. This chapter addresses these questions and will call your attention to the basic issues concerning the services that the speech/language pathologist provide.

Chapter 1

Fundamental Concepts

Before we start our discussion of clinical behavior management and the clinical process, we need to set forth some general guidelines. First of all, let us establish a more personal form of communication than that usually found in textbooks. I, the author, am writing this book for you, the reader, in an attempt to share with you my thoughts regarding the treatment of communicative disorders. The informal style the book is written in was at the request of numerous clinicians I consulted with before beginning to write. I trust the informal, conversational style and the incorporation of some humor will not distract you from the pertinence of the information.

If you are a practicing clinician, I hope that we can relate on a professional level, sharing experiences. If you are a student in training, I hope that you find my thoughts and experiences helpful as you pursue your training as a speech/language pathologist. I am not attempting to set forth new clinical approaches. I want to share with you the *Clinical Interaction Model* I have developed, which I feel will explain in a clear and concise manner what we do in our treatment programs and why we do it. The *clinical process* is an overview of the treatment program and is made up of a number of interrelated clinical processes (this is somewhat akin to a student body being made up of a number of student bodies). We will be establishing a new vocabulary related to treatment so that we can communicate clinical concepts rather than only describe clinical behaviors. Further, if we have a clearer understanding of the treatment process and the concepts that are involved, we will be able to plan more effective therapy and resolve clinical problems quicker and easier.

WHO ARE WE AND WHAT DO WE DO?

The first question we should address is "who are we?" We represent a professional group whose purpose is to "remediate" or correct communication problems. These problems are in the general areas of articulation, voice, language, and rhythm (primarily stuttering). We are a legitimate profession with a research base from which we draw information concerning the etiology and treatment of the various types of disorders with which we work. We have a well-established professional organization and numerous training programs which adhere to professional standards set forth by our national organization. We test and certify our professional people and have established ethical standards that govern our professional behavior. One of the main problems we have faced over the years is what to call ourselves.

Perhaps the problem of professional identification was best put forth by one of the leaders in our field who, when writing about our professional standards, wrote:

> In reviewing these problems, it became apparent to me that not only are our training standards vague but we have never really come to grips with the problem of defining the nature of clinical work. Before long we shall have to decide just what the professional fields of clinical speech and audiology are. Perhaps this statement seems a bit naive, but do we really know our rightful boundaries? What terms describe us: Teachers? Clinicians? Therapists? Technicians? Counselors? It was surprising to me to realize that aside from an occasional brief discussion in textbooks, our literature contains little which defines explicitly the scope of our profession.

It might surprise you to realize that this was written by Harlan Bloomer in 1956. This same problem exists in our field today. We are still not sure what the scope of our profession is or what term to use as a professional title.

In the early years of the profession we referred to ourselves as a speech correctionist but this term came into disfavor and a search began for another label. The title *speech therapist* was then coined. This term continues to be used but is not accepted by all of the profession because of semantic problems with the word *therapy*. The term has some medical overtones, inferring that therapy can only be performed with medical prescription or supervision. Although this may have been the case a number of years ago, it no longer applies. For example, the occupational therapist provides many therapeutic services without medical prescription or supervision.

The most common, and probably the most preferred, professional title used to describe us currently is *speech/language pathologist*. If we interpret this title literally, we find that the title still does not accurately describe *all* of our professional activities. The term pathology relates more specifically to the study of diseases and their manifestations. We study disorders of the communication system and we diagnose the communication disorders in our clients. So, if we stretch a point, perhaps we do function as a speech/language pathologist during our evaluations of our clients. However, this is only a small part of our total professional activities. Once we have diagnosed the particular problem, we then provide some sort of service to remediate, eliminate, or reduce the problem. Those clinical services constitute the majority of our professional time and we should acknowledge this in our professional title.

I would like to use the terms *speech clinician* and *clinician* to describe us in this book. I have not overlooked the area of language disorders, but for brevity's sake, I will use the shorter version. As long as we both understand what the terms imply, we should have no communication disorder, and, obviously, this is important in a book about communication disorders.

I would like to take this semantic problem one step further. I am not suggesting we change the professional title we have settled on, but rather to make a point regarding the type of service we provide. I would suggest that the term *teaching* accurately describes what we do with our clients in therapy. What do we actually do in the interaction we have with our clients? We *teach*! Let us view teaching as the creation of new behaviors, new concepts, or new information in a client. We do this either *directly* by presenting the new behavior, new concept, or new information, or *indirectly* by manipulating the clinical environment so that the behavior, concept, or information evolves from the environment. But, we are still teaching since we manipulated the environment in a specific way so the learning could occur.

Now, if we are teaching, we would indeed hope that the client is *learning*. This would appear to be the true test of our therapy. Is the client learning what we are attempting to teach? If we extend this concept, we would then ask the question, "Is the client learning what is expected within a reasonable period of time?" So, we are confronted with two questions regarding our therapy: How *effective* is it and how *efficient* is it? I truly believe that these are separate questions. We certainly have treatment programs that are effective in that they remediate the communication problem. However, we might ask about the efficiency of many of our programs in terms of the amount of time necessary to accomplish the clinical goals. The name of both of these games is accountability.

HOW DO WE LEARN TO DO WHAT WE DO?

Our professional learning starts in our training program. We enter a program to learn to be a speech clinician. In order to function effectively as a clinician we must have an ability to establish that mystical thing called *rapport* with our clients, technical knowledge of the various disorders, and insight into teaching strategies so that our clients can learn what we are trying to teach them. Let us discuss each of these clinical prerequisites.

What is rapport? It is impossible to define, but perhaps we can describe it. Basically, it means that there is mutual respect between the clinician and the client. It is also related to the attitude of the clinician toward therapy. If the clinician enjoys both the therapy and the client, this attitude is reflected in the therapy. It is enjoyable to both parties. The client then respects and enjoys the clinician. We can describe this phenomenon but how do we instill it in speech clinicians? A key word appears to be enthusiasm. We have all observed boring therapy. The problem here is that the clinician has no enthusiasm. Perhaps there is some truth to the old saying that clinicians are born, not made. We cannot deal further with this issue since we have yet to learn how to instill enthusiasm in a person. Let us hope that people enter the field because they enjoy it and enjoyment is the seed of enthusiasm. Also, experience is a great teacher, even in the area of developing rapport with our clients.

As for the technical knowledge, we take specialized courses in the various disorders where we learn the theories of etiology of the disorders, descriptions of the disorders, evaluative procedures, and what new behaviors, concepts, or information we need to teach the client in order to minimize or eliminate the problem. How many times have we complained that all we got was theory in our classes, nothing practical? What do we mean by practical? We learned how to evaluate the disorder and what new behaviors to introduce. We were introduced to the various etiological factors that might influence our treatment. We became intimately familiar with all aspects of a particular disorder. This information is all practical. Therapy is impossible without it. Perhaps our complaints have been misdirected. Could our complaints really be directed to the lack of practical information on how to actually do therapy? Where do we get the information pertinent to the clinical interaction in the clinic room?

LEARNING "HOW" TO DO THERAPY

How do we learn the HOW of therapy? We learn from our clinical observations, our clinical methods course, our clinical experiences, and from conferences with our clinical supervisors. Let us discuss each of these. Clinical observations are usually assigned to students early in their training program, primarily so that they can see what the profession is all about. These are very general observations since, at this point in their training, the students do not know the field. Other observation assignments may be made later in training in some training programs. In this case, the first observations are to get a general idea of the role of the speech clinician in the clinic room and the later observations are to provide the student with an opportunity to study the clinical interaction in therapy; the therapy procedure. It is probably during these observations that the student clinician begins to seek *recipes* for treating the various types of disorders. Since they do not understand the therapy process at this point in their training, they attempt to formulate a standard approach to each disorder based on what they have observed.

The material covered in clinical methods courses or their equivalents varies widely. In some courses the HOW of therapy is discussed and perhaps even demonstrated. The problem instructors face in presenting the HOW of therapy is the lack of any published material on this aspect of therapy. This book has been written to fill this gap. In any event, the students do gain insight into the therapy process in these classes in preparation for their forthcoming clinical experience.

We now move into the third and fourth factors, clinical experience and conferences with the supervisor. It is at this time that a clinical team is formed, the student clinician and the clinical supervisor. After the client is assigned to the student and the client's files have been reviewed, the clinical team has a conference to plan the therapy. Lesson plans are written and reviewed. The supervisor's main job at this time is to get the clinician to give up the recipes and actually plan a therapy program for the individual client. This continues even after the clinician has started to work with the client. The clinician has no experience to draw on, only the information gained in observations, the clinical methods course, and the first few conferences with the supervisor. Recipes offer security blankets for floundering clinicians. The conferences with the supervisor are concerned with evaluating the therapy that has been done and with planning where the therapy will go in the next several sessions. Unfortunately, the evaluation of the therapy is "after the fact," the mistakes have already been made. At first these conferences are somewhat limited in their effectiveness because the clinician does not have the extensive clinical vocabulary and grasp of clinical concepts that the supervisor has. The clinician sometimes has great difficulty in "catching on" to what the supervisor is trying to teach. However, as the clinician gains clinical experience, the conference becomes more effective since the clinician is learning clinical concepts and a more extensive clinical vocabulary. Eventually, the student clinician completes the clinical requirements of the training program (sometimes to the wonderment of the supervisor) and, upon graduation, is ready to function professionally as a speech clinician. We now move into another phase of learning the HOW of therapy through clinical experience: "on-the-job training."

Let us look at this positively. A good clinician never stops learning to do therapy. There are always new types of clients, new challenges, new approaches. It is impossible for a training program to prepare the student for every possible type of client and clinical setting. We simply leave one learning environment and enter another. But, let us hope that we made all of our serious clinical errors during our training while we were able to consult with our clinical supervisor.

Earlier in our profession, training programs had not developed the extensive supervisory skills that are found in the training programs today. These techniques took many years to evolve. Clinicians who were trained in the 1940s and the 1950s did not have the extensive supervision opportunities available in today's training programs. At that time, much of the learning of clinical skills occurred through trial and error with little opportunity to consult with a supervisor. The clinical history of our field is important so the clinicians of today do not repeat all of the clinical errors that others have made in the past.

Allow me to share with you my experience as I attempted to learn HOW to do therapy. Perhaps this will give you more insight into the need for a clinical history. I started my training by observing other students in my program doing the therapy. These student clinicians were one year ahead of me and many of them were working with their first client. I observed very carefully and made notes on what I *thought* was transpiring. The only person that I had to discuss my observations with was the student clinician and other student observers. What was I attempting to learn through my observations? I supposedly had much of the technical information, but I needed to understand the teaching strategies used by the student clinician. My conferences with the student clinician were what is commonly referred to as "the blind leading the blind."

After relatively few hours of observation of other students doing therapy, the moment of truth arrived. I was enrolled in a clinical practicum course and, shortly thereafter, received notification that I had been assigned a client. Following the initial unique combination of thrill and total panic I went to the clinical files and reviewed what the previous clinicians had written. My client's file was extremely thick with report after report from student clinicians that the client had trained. These were the truly frightening clients since, after training so many generations of student clinicians, they knew more about therapy than the student clinicians. Having reviewed the client's file, I then discussed my new client with those other poor souls who were attempting to get their courage up to meet their first client. Misery loves company.

Following a brief conference with my clinical supervisor, I wrote up my first, but definitely not my last, clinical lesson plan. How I struggled with that first attempt to figure out what to do for an entire therapy period. I tried to plan what I would say to the client the first time we met. What would I say to the parents? How would I establish that mysterious thing called rapport that everyone talked about but could not define? Would I like my client? Would my client like me? Anxiety! This is when I learned the real meaning of the term.

My first client's name was Gary. He was a 9-year-old, language retarded, hyperactive, destructive child. In our first meeting I called upon my vast reserve of observational experience (about 30 hours) and found, much to my chagrin, that my observations did not include a client of this nature. Undaunted, I plunged ahead with my clinical activities that I had so carefully prepared in my lesson plan. As you might expect, the first 30-minute clinical meeting was a total disaster. I ignored Gary and he ignored me. I was so preoccupied with following my lesson plan that I was oblivious to the fact that Gary was paying attention to everything in the therapy room, except me. My lesson plan was very efficient. I finished the entire plan in 15 minutes. I will not go into the morbid details of how the remaining 15 minutes were spent. The only bright side to this clinical experience was that, in the future, my therapy could only improve. As I look back, I hope that Gary eventually learned as much from me as I did from him. I also hope he survived the multitudes of clinicians he trained. My clinical supervisor attempted to point out all of the things that were wrong in the therapy session but there was just too much to cover. She struggled through this client with me, but most of the time I did not understand the points she was attempting to make with me. I did not have either the clinical vocabulary or the clinical concepts I needed to fully appreciate the guidance she was trying to give me. Unfortunately, these conferences were few and far between and always after I had already made the mistakes.

In retrospect, I think I know what I wanted to teach Gary, but I did not understand the clinical process. I did not know *HOW* to teach him. I only knew what I had seen. I did not understand it but I could *imitate* it if all of the conditions from my observations were the same in my therapy. Realistically, this just does not happen. Every client is different, as are the interactions between clients and clinicians. My first clinical experience could be used as a classical example of how *not* to do therapy! If there was anything I could have done wrong that I did not do wrong, it was simply an oversight on my part.

The value of clinical observations early in my training program was quite limited. Yes, I saw things going on that I could repeat in another clinical situation, but this was imitation of a process, not the understanding of the process. Competent clinical planning could not occur since I did not understand the clinical process itself. This type of learning is akin to learning neurosurgery through observation, without having any background in neuroanatomy or neurophysiology. Before I observed ongoing therapy I should have been made aware of the basic principles that are involved so that I could understand what I was seeing.

THERAPY SHOULD BE LAWFUL, NOT AWFUL

In my years as a teacher, clinician, and supervisor I have seen many examples of "awful" therapy. Before we describe "awful" therapy, let us apply the "OP Rule." This means that all "awful" therapy is done by "Other People." "Awful" therapy is boring. Both the clinician and the client are bored. There is no rapport between the clinician and the client. The therapy is not planned, it is not organized, and there is little interaction between the clinician and the client. Neither the clinician nor the client are aware of the clinical goal and the therapy has no purpose. Even the clinical activities have no purpose since there is no goal. Everything appears to be occurring at random. Obviously this list could go on and on but I will let you fill in other factors.

Therapy involves both the teaching skills of the clinician and the learning skills of the client. In order to develop teaching skills, the clinician must understand *how* and *why* people learn. With this information, teaching strategies can be developed that are both effective and efficient. The interaction between the clinician and the client should not be a random learning experience that occurs by chance or by luck. It should be guided by specific principles of learning. If these basic principles are understood and used in clinical planning, the treatment process becomes a predictable interaction with a predictable outcome. Also, if a clinical procedure is planned according to these principles but, due to an unforeseen factor, the procedure is not effective, the principles will indicate where the problem is and how it may be resolved. This is our professional challenge—to be able to plan an appropriate and effective clinical program for our clients, regardless of the type of communication disorder manifested, and to make sure that the program is time efficient. This is a professional obligation as well as a moral obligation. Our first task to increase our clinical efficiency is to organize therapy into a logical sequence of events.

The Treatment Sequence

As we move into the treatment of communication disorders let us consider what the steps of our treatment program are. For the sake of brevity and clarity, I refer to the speech clinician as "she" and the client as "he" for the remainder of the book. In our discussion, the five steps of treatment are:

1. *Evaluating the client.* When we do a diagnostic evaluation of a client, we are gathering data for a number of reasons. We need to know what the particular problem is and an indication of the severity of the problem. We also try to determine the reason the problem exists since this will influence the type of treatment program we are going to plan for the client. One of the most important things we look for is evidence of some organic involvement such as structural deviation or neurological involvement. If there is an *organic* base to the problem, this must be considered when we decide what our clinical goals will be. Another factor we must be concerned with is the cognitive level of the client since this has direct bearing on how we will approach the client in terms of teaching the new behavior. This calls for either formal or informal assessment of the client's cognitive skills, attitudes, motivation for therapy, and environmental factors, to name a few. There are still other factors we are concerned with in the evaluation, but they are too numerous to mention here, particularly since we are not directly concerned with the evaluative process in this book. However, you should be aware of the importance of this data gathering process as it relates to your clinical planning. Our technical information is vital here.

2. *Determining behavior change goals.* After we have gathered as much information as we need regarding the client and the communication problem, we can then determine which behavior we want to change and what the behavior change goal is to be. The behavior change goal is dependent on what we have found in our evaluation. The type of disorder, the severity of the disorder, the presence of an organic factor, the cognitive level of the client, and other factors are all considered when we determine what behavior we are going to concentrate on and what the behavior change goal is. It is at this point that we again call upon the technical

information from our specialized courses to assist us in making this decision.

3. ***Getting the new behavior to occur.*** Having decided what behavior to work on and what the behavior change goal is, we then proceed to teach the new behavior. It is at this point in the treatment program that therapy begins. Prior to this we have been involved in testing and planning phases of treatment. Now we are entering the teaching and learning phases of treatment. This is the beginning of the clinical process, the HOW of therapy. We must now introduce the behavior to the client in such a way that it can be learned and performed independent of prompts or cues.

4. ***Habituating the new behavior.*** Once the new behavior has been learned in the clinical environment, it must be habituated in that environment. The new behavior must occur correctly and without any influence from the clinician. It must be stabilized in the clinic room before it can be generalized into the client's natural speaking environments.

5. ***Generalizing the new behavior.*** Therapy is not completed until the new behavior is occurring automatically in all of the client's talking environments. The speech clinician is still involved in this last step of therapy, although her clinical activities will change.

During my early years of experience as a speech clinician, I felt the most secure in the first two steps of the treatment program. As a profession, we have established reliable and valid evaluative procedures for all of the communicative disorders. I would include here diagnostic treatment where the final decision regarding the diagnosis of the communicative disorder comes only after some treatment procedures have been tested. I was also quite comfortable with determining the behavior change goals of my clients. This information was included in the courses I took in my training program and is also to be found in almost any textbook.

I felt much less secure with the third step of treatment, where I entered the therapy aspect of the treatment program. I knew many techniques, such as the *stimulus method, moto-kinesthetics,* and *providing models,* but I did not understand the dynamics involved. And I found that I did not have a source to go to for help. It was even difficult to discuss this aspect of therapy with other clinicians since we did not have a vocabulary to describe the teaching process. This was the HOW of therapy and I had to learn it through trial and error. I later found that this was also the part of the total treatment program that I could not teach to my students so they would not repeat all of my clinical errors.

The fourth step, habituation, did not present insurmountable problems. With drill work and conversation I was able to get new behaviors to occur consistently and correctly in the clinic room. I may not have been very efficient but I always managed to stabilize the behavior in the clinical environment.

I felt the least secure with the last step of the treatment program, generalization. From my discussions with other clinicians, I found that I was not alone in my insecurity. It appeared that this was the major problem that most clinicians faced, and this was the step in the treatment program that was the least discussed in our literature. We were able to create the new speech behaviors in the clinic room successfully but had difficulty in getting the behavior to occur naturally in other speaking environments. This last step in treatment was questionable both in terms of effectiveness and efficiency, and this same problem continues to plague the profession today.

THE CLINICAL PROCESS

The treatment of communication disorders has been set forth as five rather distinct steps. Let us now further divide our treatment program into two aspects of therapy, the *evaluative–planning process* and the *clinical process*. The evaluative–planning process includes the evaluation of the client and determining behavior change goals. The clinical process consists of getting the behavior to occur, habituating the new behavior, and generalizing the new behavior.

We discuss the clinical process in this book. This is not to say that the evaluative–planning process is of lesser importance, but that it represents a prelude to therapy rather than the clinical intervention itself. Let us not forget, however, that the therapy plan that we adopt for the clinical process is totally dependent on the information we gather and the decisions we make in the evaluative–planning process.

Finally, regardless of how well we are prepared for therapy, we must consider the effects of certain laws of nature on the clinical process. We cannot prevent their occurrence but if we understand them we can minimize their effects. After much deliberation and study I have set forth these laws which are to be found in Appendix A. I would recommend that you study them before proceeding with the book.

Synopsis

Having established that our contracts with our clients should be a teaching/learning experience, we need to understand the dynamics of the clinical situation. Our clinical interactions are governed by principles and concepts. If we understand them and carefully incorporate them into our therapy, our therapy becomes more effective and more efficient. This predictable and lawful interaction can be manipulated by the clinician in many ways to adjust it to the demands of each unique situation. This chapter concerns the *Clinical Interaction Model* which sets forth the operational aspects of this clinical interaction. This model will assist the clinician in planning therapy and resolving clinical problems when they arise.

Chapter 2

Cognitive Behavior Therapy: A Model

THE CORE OF THERAPY

Now that we know what we do, let us talk about how we do it. Essentially, what we are doing is teaching the client new speech behaviors, attitudes, or beliefs. The effectiveness of our therapy is dependent on how well the client learns what we are attempting to teach. So the most important ingredient of our therapy is the client's learning. How does the client learn? There are many theories and concepts regarding human learning, but there is no single one that satisfactorily explains all of the learning that goes on in the clinical environment. We cannot go into a detailed presentation of each and every learning theory or concept, but we will briefly discuss some of the basic assumptions and concepts of those theories that are of particular interest to speech clinicians. In that we are limited to such brief discussions, I would highly recommend that you do additional reading in this area. The more information you have about the various theories and concepts, the better you will understand your therapy. I would refer you to the Recommended Readings section where many references are listed. Since some of these references are quite theoretical and abstract, I would suggest you start with the book by Lefrancois (1972). He covers most of the learning theories and concepts and his humorous approach makes the reading easy. I would next suggest the book edited by Perkins (1982) which applies these theories and concepts to our therapy. Further references are also available from a variety of sources in any library. Now let us take a brief look at some of the more common learning theories and concepts that are used by the speech clinician.

LEARNING THEORIES AND CONCEPTS

Classical Conditioning

In classical conditioning, responses are elicited by stimuli. If the stimulus is not present, the conditioned response will not occur. In the conditioning process, a bond is established between the stimulus and the response so that each time the stimulus is presented, the response occurs. The name we associate with this form of conditioning is Pavlov. He conditioned a dog to salivate (response) when a bell was rung (stimulus). This concept is clearly demonstrated by the Wizard in Figure 1.

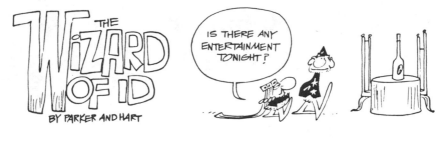

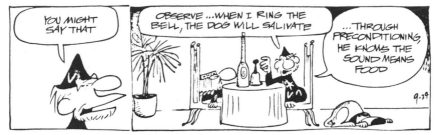

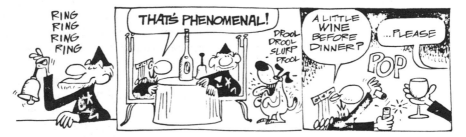

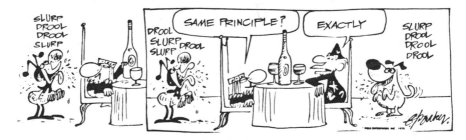

FIGURE 1
Wizard of Id

Just as with the work of Pavlov, the dog has been conditioned to associate the ringing of a bell with food. So, when the bell rings, the dog drools and slurps. The jester? Same principle? Exactly!

A treatment method has been devised which is related to classical conditioning. It is Systematic Desensitization. If a client has been conditioned to respond to a stimulus with fear, anxiety, and tension, he is taught an alternative response, relaxation. The stimulus is then presented in graduated steps, starting with the presentation of the least disturbing aspect of the stimulus. The process continues as the client maintains his relaxation, until the client can remain relaxed even when the stimulus is presented at full strength. Clinical application is found primarily in the treatment of phobias or feared situations which inconvenience a person. The procedure can also be used with stutterers who have fear of talking on the telephone. When the stutterer is relaxed and fluent, the telephone is gradually presented as the stutterer maintains his relaxation and fluency. If the stutterer tenses and begins to stutter, the hierarchy (look at it, touch it, pick it up, etc.) is temporarily halted until the stutterer regains his relaxation. The presentation then resumes until tension is present again. The procedure is continued until the stutterer is "desensitized" to the telephone. Many universities have desensitization programs to assist students who have uncontrollable anxiety associated with tests (my students highly recommend such a program).

Operant Conditioning

With regard to operant or instrumental conditioning, the response is not directly related to a stimulus. The response is emitted rather than elicited. Also, the learning experience is dependent on the consequence of the response. If the consequence is positive for the person, the response has been reinforced and the probability that it will occur again is increased. If the consequence is negative, the response has been punished and the probability of future occurrence is decreased. In Figure 2 you will see that Ziggy is learning to respond through reinforcement.

Chances are that when Ziggy goes back into the Dog Trainer's office he will *fetch* the ashtray, since this behavior was reinforced. Will he also hand the Dog Trainer $20 each time he enters the office? This will depend on how much he likes the "Doggie Yum Yums."

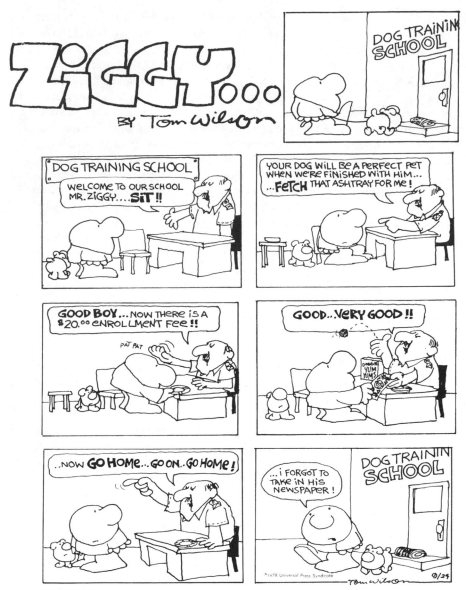

FIGURE 2
Ziggy

As was just mentioned, we also learn things through punishment. It is a bit different in that, when our behavior is punished, we tend not to perform it again in order to avoid the punishment. This is a strong form of learning as you will see in Figure 3.

FOR BETTER OR WORSE

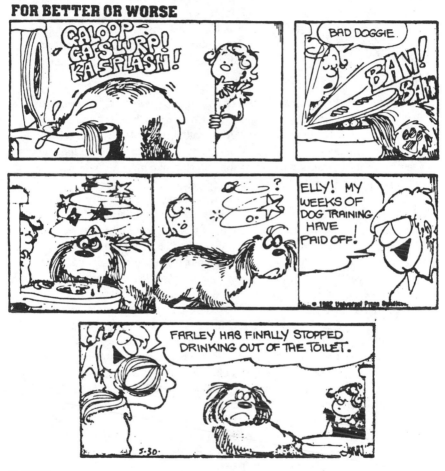

FIGURE 3
For Better or Worse

Will Farley drink out of the toilet again? Not if he can help it. He will avoid this since he *knows* that when he does, he gets banged on the head. Farley may be a dog, but he is not stupid. This is called learning the hard way.

The clinical applications of operant conditioning are found in all aspects of treatment of general behavior disorders. Some programs are based on reinforcing appropriate behaviors, some on punishing inappropriate behaviors, and others use a combination of reinforcement and punishment. This clinical approach is widely used by speech clinicians in all forms of therapy. We encourage correct speech behaviors to occur through reinforcement and discourage the occurrence of incorrect speech behaviors through punishment.

Modeling

One of the most common forms of learning to perform a new behavior is by watching and or listening to someone perform the behavior and then attempting to reproduce the behavior. According to Bandura (1969) this is referred to as modeling, imitation, observational learning, identification, copying, vicarious learning, social facilitation, contagion, or role playing. We will use the term *modeling* for this form of learning.

Consider learning such activities as driving a car, swimming, or operating a computer. These activities could all be learned by trial and error or learned in gradual steps (shaping) but these forms of learning would not be very efficient. Think of what would have happened if you had learned to drive a car strictly by trial and error. Can you imagine the costs for repairing not only your car but all of the cars you had run into? By the time you had learned to drive you would not be able to buy insurance and the local police would have barred you from the streets. Your learning to drive would have been more effective if you had a model you could use as a pattern for your own behavior (it is always better if the model is not provided by the parents of the beginning driver since this usually results in negative emotions and even worse language). When a model is presented, the learner has the goal behavior clearly set forth and the randomness of his behavioral performance is greatly reduced. With a model, most of his behavioral performances are goal oriented.

It is important to recognize that many modeling–learning approaches assume that there is reward associated with the performance of the imitated behavior. This reward could be either a direct reward for behavioral performance or the intrinsic reward of successfully imitating the model. We will assume this view of learning through modeling.

Modeling is an important factor in understanding how children learn to talk. It explains why children learn to speak with the same accent or dialect as their parents. Speech clinicians have used this form of learning from the very beginning of the profession. It is reflected in the comment of one clinician who tells her clients to "listen and watch, think about it, and then try it." We set forth the speech goal for the client by modeling it so that the client not only knows what is expected of him, but he also has seen and/or heard it performed and has a better idea of how to recreate it.

Motor Learning

Motor skills are frequently referred to as *perceptual–motor skills*. This terminology is used to emphasize the coordination between sensory input (perception) and the performance of the behavior (motor skill). The concept of motor skill learning is typically applied to eye–hand coordination skills such as handling a tennis racket or swinging a golf club. In most references you will find that speech–motor learning is excluded from perceptual–motor skill learning and included as part of verbal learning. However, the concepts involved in perceptual–motor skill learning are directly applicable to our therapy.

This is a complex form of learning and concerns the learning of specific motor skills. First of all we need to define what we mean by a skill. Generally it refers to a chain or sequence of motor responses (muscular movements) that are learned through the coordination of various sensory and motor systems in the body. The skill is then organized into complex response patterns. When we apply these principles to learning motor movements involved in speech, the primary sensory systems that are involved in this learning experience are the visual and the auditory systems. An example of application of this learning system to speech would be learning a consonant/vowel/consonant (CVC) syllable by listening to and watching a person produce it. The CVC syllable represents a sequence of muscular movements involving several motor systems (the tongue, jaw, lips, etc.). This CVC syllable is then organized into a complex response pattern, the client's speech.

Let us consider the sequence involved in learning a new motor skill. According to Fitts (1962), there are three phases involved: cognitive, fixation, and autonomous. In the first phase the "teacher" provides information about the new behavior and models it. The "learner" then thinks about the information and the model and develops a plan of how he will perform the behavior. When he has completed his planning, he then attempts the behavior. This continues until the behavior is relatively stable. The second phase, fixation, consists of the learner practicing the new behavior until there are no errors in the behavior. In the final phase, autonomous, the speed of production is increased to the point where it is functional as a part of a larger behavioral unit. This sequence reflects what occurs when we teach the client a new speech behavior. We provide a model and information about the behavior. The client then thinks about it and forms a plan of how to imitate the model. He then attempts to imitate the model as he perceives it. When the model has been accurately imitated we move into the next phase of therapy where the behavior is practiced until it occurs consistently with no errors. The next step in therapy is to increase the speed of production of the new behavior so that it fits into the larger behavioral unit, the client's speech.

Cognitive Learning

There are many theories and concepts which could be classified under the heading of cognitive learning. In essence, these theories and concepts believe that the "thinking" or cognitive process of the individual is involved in such activities as perception, problem solving through insight, decision making, processing information, and comprehension. Of all of the various aspects of cognition, the most important to the speech clinician are memory and problem solving.

There are two types of memory, long term and short term. Long-term memory concerns the retention of information for long periods of time. This type of information is maintained since it is rehearsed often, and includes items such as your name and telephone number. Long-term memory of a person's age fades after he/she reaches 39 years of age. When information is not rehearsed or used, it is forgotten. Think back to your class in anatomy and see what information you remember. You will recall or remember only that information you have recalled or used as a clinician. Or, take a class where you crammed, not to learn the information but just to get a passing grade in the course; you probably do not remember any of the information or, perhaps, even the name of the course. This latter example leads us to short-term memory.

Short-term memory consists of bits of information that we retain only for a short period of time since it is not needed over an extended time period. We use our short-term memory to remember a telephone number we have looked up long enough so that we can dial it. We also use it, or should use it, at parties where we are introduced to people and remember their names only for the duration of the party. This type of information is not vital to our survival so we do not commit it to our long-term memory system.

Both forms of memory are important to therapy. If we teach a client a new behavior or concept, we expect him to remember it over an extended period of time. If the client does not have long-term memory we have great difficulty with our therapy. These clients come into therapy each time as though it were the first session. Clinical progress is dependent on long-term memory.

Short-term memory has a more immediate impact on our therapy. We give our clients instructions such as, "Put the spoon in the cup and hand me the knife," or we ask them to repeat messages such as "Repeat after me, 'I found a fat frog.'" If a client cannot retain this information long enough to perform the task, therapy is going to be extremely difficult.

The other aspect of cognitive learning that has an impact on our therapy is problem solving through insight. When people are confronted with a problem, something they do not understand, they compare it with their memories of similar experiences, information they have, and other cognitive resources. In other words, they think about the problem in terms of their own knowledge, memories, and experiences. If their thinking results in a solution to the problem, it occurs very quickly. Suddenly, the solution is very clear and all of the factors involved are obvious. The best way to explain this is to let you experience it. Please look at the "word games" that follow. Each of the three games represents a term or phrase that a speech clinician would use. The solution to the games lies in the relationship between the words, the spacing of the words, or some such factor. Do not take the words at face value. See if you can do some problem solving by insight.

1. PAL ATE
2. PITUPCH
3. ARTIK, ARTIK, ARTIK

I do hope that you had some success in finding a solution to the word games. If not, you are going to have to look at Appendix B for the solutions. You will also find there a few more word games for you to solve

The gaining of insight is very important to our therapy. We confront our clients with many problems to which they must find solutions. We present them with a variety of stimuli which they must integrate and gain insight into before they can utilize the information. We present them with a model of a sound, give them some information about how it is made, and then we expect them to be able to produce it. They must integrate all of this information and achieve insight into the relationships before they can respond appropriately. We give clients numerous rules concerning phonology and expect this to influence their speech production. However, there will be no influence until the clients gain insight into the relationship between the rules we give them and their speech. This is a part of verbal comprehension, the complete understanding of what is presented on a verbal level. It involves not only understanding the individual words, but also their relationships and the concepts that they convey. Perhaps we achieve comprehension and understanding only as the client gains insight into the problems we present to him.

ESTABLISHING A CLINICAL VOCABULARY

As I mentioned earlier, one of the main problems we have when we discuss therapy is the lack of a vocabulary which communicates clinical concepts. We are currently limited to a vocabulary that describes only our clinical behaviors. Before we go further in the discussion of the clinical process, it is important that we establish a clinical vocabulary so that we can communicate on a concept level.

The Cognitive Behavioral Approach

The cognitive aspect of our *cognitive behavior therapy* is eclectic in nature in that it utilizes concepts from a number of learning paradigms. The cognitive behavior approach to therapy may appear to be unique in that it combines cognitive learning with noncognitive conditioning procedures and, to some, this may seem to be a contradiction. But, the client's cognitions cannot be prevented or ignored. They are a part of any treatment procedure, regardless of the intent of the theoretic approach. Our approach is not unique. It is a reflection of the "Cognitive Behavior Modification" movement started by Meichenbaum in the late 1970s.

In getting a new behavior to occur, we use a number of techniques that depend on the client's cognitions. We may model the new behavior but the client must be aware of it, perceive it, think about it, and then shift it from the abstract perception to the concrete production. We may physically guide the client's tongue in the production of a sound. Again, the client must be cognitively involved in applying this information when he attempts to make the correct production of the sound. In this context, the client is constantly involved in therapy on a cognitive level.

We must also look at cognition from the standpoint of the cognitive involvement of the clinician. This is not meant as a facetious remark. If the clinician is performing her therapy in a reflexive manner, she is probably not deeply involved on a cognitive level. However, good therapy calls for the clinician to be totally involved on a cognitive level; evaluating the client's responses, determining an appropriate response to the client's behavior, changing the clinical strategy if the client fails to respond or comprehend. And, let us not forget that the clinician must be aware of the client's attitudes, emotions, feelings, and needs. These play an important part in therapy and the clinician must take them into consideration not only in planning a treatment program but also as treatment progresses. In some instances, the treatment program might focus on these factors, a matter discussed in detail in Chapter 8. In any event, there must be a total commitment of the thinking process to the ongoing clinical interaction. Effective and efficient therapy is hard work on the part of the clinician as well as the client.

Special Semantic Problems

Any attempt to bridge the gap between theory and therapy results in the compromise of one or both positions. In our cognitive behavioral approach, both are compromised. However, I have attempted to make the compromises as palatable as possible for both the theoretician and the practitioner. Further, attempts to simplify complex systems often leads to oversimplification. This is an inherent problem with our cognitive behavioral approach. I can only hope that, as you and I gain more clinical experience and deeper insight into principles and concepts of learning, we expand and fill in the clinical framework presented in this book.

There are several terms we will be using that need to be discussed before you read their definitions. The terms *reinforce* and *punish* often cause confusion and misunderstanding, particularly the term punish. In much of the literature concerning operant conditioning, the terms *reward* and *penalty* are used as synonyms for reinforce and punish. We will use these terms since they are much clearer in meaning to most people. This can be extremely important in those clinical environments where we are communicating with other people such as teachers, occupational therapists, physical therapists, physicians, or clinical aids who may not have a clear understanding of the terms reinforce and punish. Further, the term penalize seems to have a less negative connotation than does the term punish. Depending on the agency where the clinical services are offered, this could be very important.

When we use reward or penalty, we set up different cognitive sets or mental attitudes in our clients. When we apply a reward, the client has a positive attitude and repeats his rewarded behavior in order to get more rewards. However, when we apply a penalty, the client's attitude becomes negative and he changes his behavior in order to escape from or avoid the penalty. We need terms to describe these different attitudes the client might have in therapy. This is important since we will be discussing clinical strategies to purposely create these different attitudes. However, there do not appear to be standard terms that we can use here. If we turn to clinical terminology, we find that many clinicians use the term *motivation* to describe the client's attitude toward therapy. However, motivation can be interpreted as a client being motivated to achieve rewards or to avoid penalty.

Two other terms that are related to these client attitudes are *approach* and *avoidance*. The positive mental attitude is approach and the negative is avoidance. The positive mental attitude leads to approach behavior to achieve more rewards while the negative mental attitude leads to the avoidance of penalty.

We will combine the terms into *approach motivation* and *avoidance motivation* and use these terms to describe the two attitudinal states we are discussing. When a behavior is followed by a positive consequence (reward), the client develops approach motivation which results in the behavior being performed more often. When a behavior is followed by a negative consequence (penalty), the client develops avoidance motivation which results in the behavior being performed less often.

We are now ready to create our clinical vocabulary. In that the cognitive behavioral approach is eclectic, terms from several different learning paradigms are used. Read the following definitions carefully since some definitions include examples related to our cognitive behavioral approach. The definitions will be expanded in later chapters and clinical examples will be provided to futher clarify the terms and the concepts they represent.

Clinical Vocabulary

Behavior. A behavior is anything a person does. Overt behaviors are actions or movements that can be observed. Covert behaviors are thoughts or feelings that cannot be observed but are still considered behaviors. There is a concept known as the "dead man" rule which indicates that anything a living person can do that a "dead man" cannot do is a behavior. This should give us room to operate.

Behaviors have three characteristics which we will be concerned with; their frequency of occurrence, their strength or intensity when they occur, and their duration once they do occur. We will be manipulating these characteristics as we move through the clinical process.

Stimulus (S). A stimulus is anything which attracts a person's attention. It may be something inside the person such as a headache or something in his/her external environment such as objects in a room. We will not view a stimulus as an event which elicits a behavior but rather as an event which prompts or cues a behavior to occur. The behavior may be either overt or covert.

Response (R). A response is the reaction a person has to a stimulus, a behavior. Responses include thinking about the stimulus, looking at an object in a room, imitating a speech behavior presented by the clinician, and rewarding a client for a correct behavior.

Antecedent event. An antecedent event precedes the response: that is, the stimulus that prompts or cues a response to occur is an antecedent event.

Modeling. Modeling is the demonstration of behavior. We show the clients what we want them to do. This could include such diverse behaviors as the production of the [r] sound, maintaining eye contact, opening the jaw further during speech, slowing down the rate of speech, or using the correct syntax. This is the demonstration of the behavior change goal so that our clients know what we expect them to do.

Information. In our contact with the clients we can either provide for the client or request from the client two types of information. First, we can provide *behavioral* information that is concerned with the behavior we are attempting to teach. This type of information might include such things as telling the client to prolong the vowel when attempting to slow down the rate of speech, or to hold the teeth closer together when attempting to make the [s] sound. We can also request the client to repeat what we have said to him to make sure he understood us.

Second, we can provide *general* information. This might include a description of our therapy, therapy goals, and information to change attitudes or emotions. Again, we might ask the client to repeat what we have told him to determine his perception of what we said. We can also ask the client for information concerning his attitudes, emotions, and feelings regarding his communicative disorder. This is the basis for any counseling we might have to do with the client.

Guidance. Another term for guidance would be *prompt*. There are four types of guidance that we use in therapy. We give *verbal* guidance in the form of hints or cues about the behavior. *Gestural* guidance includes those gestures we make to prompt or cue a behavior to occur. We also use *environmental* guidance when we manipulate the environment so that it prompts the behavior, such as showing the client a picture. Finally, we use *physical* guidance where we actually touch the client to assist in the performance of a behavior.

Contingent event. An event which follows the response is contingent. Basically, this means either a pleasant event (reward) or an unpleasant event (penalty) that occurs immediately after the response.

Reward (R+). Reward is the same as reinforcement. It signifies the positive event which occurs after a behavior is performed. If the event is truly rewarding to the client, the chances of the behavior occurring again are increased.

Penalty (P). Penalty is the same as punishment. It signifies the negative event which occurs after a behavior is performed. If the event is truly penalizing to the client, the chances of the behavior occurring again are decreased.

Extinguish. When reward for a behavior is withheld, the behavior will extinguish. It will no longer occur since the reward is no longer presented and the behavior no longer has a purpose. However, if the behavior has become self-rewarding it will continue to occur since it is no longer dependent on an external reward.

Reward schedule. When we use the term reward schedule, we are referring to how often we reward behavior. A continuous schedule means that we reward every occurrence of a behavior. This provides fast learning but the behavior is not very stable and will have a tendency to cease to occur when the reward is removed. With an intermittent schedule we reward on a more random basis. There are two types of intermittent systems. In the "ratio" system, either fixed or variable, the reward is given based on the number of times the behavior has occurred. In the "interval" system, the determining factor for reward is time. The intermittent schedule is not as efficient for learning a behavior but makes the behavior very stable and the behavior will have a tendency to continue to occur even after the reward is removed.

Approach motivation. Approach motivation represents the mental attitude of the client where the focus of therapy is on rewards. He will perform the behavior being rewarded more often in order to get more rewards.

Avoidance motivation. Avoidance motivation represents the mental attitude of the client where the focus of therapy is on penalties. He will perform the behavior being penalized less often in order to avoid the penalty.

Shaping. Shaping is the process of creating a *new* behavior in a client. As behaviors more closely approximate the target behavior, they are rewarded and through this process the new behavior is gradually shaped.

Significant others. Significant others are the people who are very important in the client's life. It may be the client's parents, foster parents, wife, husband, or close friend.

Token economy. When the client is initially rewarded with tokens, such as poker chips, which he can turn in at some later time for a more meaningful reward, this is referred to as a token economy.

Stimulus control. Stimuli can be manipulated in several ways. They can be gradually presented, gradually withdrawn, increased in number, decreased in number, or their prompting role changed. This is stimulus control.

Fading. Fading is the gradual removal of a stimulus. Remember that when we reward a client, the reward is a stimulus to the client and can be gradually withdrawn (faded).

THE CLINICIAN/CLIENT INTERACTION

The Relationships

The dynamics of the interaction between the clinician and the client can best be viewed as a continuous series of transactions. These transactions are basically of two types: "small talk" and "clinical." Small talk is used to establish rapport or, in many instances, because the clinician forgot to plan therapy. Since the small talk transactions seem to come naturally to most clinicians, especially when they are not prepared for therapy, we will concern ourselves with the clinical transactions. These transactions can best be illustrated by using some of the terms we have just defined and showing them in proper sequential order. The first half of a transaction would appear like this:

$$\underline{S - O - R}$$

This equation represents the clinician presenting the stimulus (S) to the client (O = organism/cognition). The clinician might be modeling the correct production of the [k] sound. As the client hears and sees the model (perceives it), he will think about it (cognition) before he attempts to imitate it. When he does make his attempt to imitate it we have his response (R). We have now completed one half of the transaction. The clinician must now respond to the client, so we will expand the diagram.

$$(S - O - R/\underline{S - O - R})$$

The first half of the diagram remains the same but now we see that the response (R) of the client becomes the stimulus (S) for the clinician. As she hears and sees the client's response she must make some very important decisions and then respond to the client. This completes the first transaction of ongoing therapy, the first of a continuing series of transactions between the clinician and the client. To continue the interaction between the clinician and the client we must again expand our diagram.

$$(S - O - R/S - O - R)(\underline{S - O - R}$$

Now, it the clinician's turn to provide another S that will start the next transaction. When she evaluates the client's last response she decides where the transaction should go and what she is going to say. Let us consider an example of this. In the first transaction, the client is attending and has responded with a sound that is close to the correct [k] sound. The clinician's response to the client's [k] production might be a reward such as "That was a good sound." She then starts the second transaction by saying, "Now, let's try it again. Listen— [k]." The stimulus is then the repeating of the model of the [k] sound. The cycle starts over again with the client seeing and hearing the sound, thinking about it, and then trying it. This second response is another stimulus for the clinician to respond to. We must expand the diagram one more step.

$$(S - O - R/S - O - R)(S - O - R/\underline{S - O - R})$$

The clinician now makes her decisions and responds to the second attempt. We have two transactions completed. Perhaps it would be easier if we could visualize these clinical transactions in a circular form such as that illustrated in Figure 4.

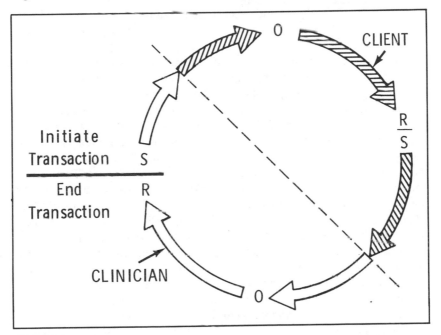

FIGURE 4
Clinical Transaction Diagram. The clinical transaction is initiated by the clinician's stimulus (S). The client thinks about the stimulus (O) and then responds (R). The client's response is the stimulus (S) for the clinician. She evaluates the client's stimulus (O) and then responds (R). This constitutes one clinical transaction. The clinician's next stimulus (S) initiates the next transaction.

Visualize these transactions as continuing around the circle: one time around for each succeeding transaction. Therapy, then, is like a string of beads, with each transaction building on and following the previous transaction. Each stimulus from the clinician is dependent on her evaluation of the client's performance in the previous transaction. Let us consider an example of the two transactions we discussed earlier. We start the initial transaction with:

S—clinician modeling [k];
O—client perceiving and thinking about the model;
R—client produces approximation to [k];
S—sound production for clinician;
O—evaluation by the clinician;
R—clinician says, "That was very good."
(This is the stimulus for approach motivation)
(End first transaction)

S—clinician says, "Make the sound again—[k]";
O—client perceives and thinks about model;
R—client produces approximation to [k];
S—sound production for clinician;
O—evaluation by clinician;
R—clinician responds accordingly.
(End second transaction)

Clinical Testing

One of the most important factors to remember is that these transactions between the clinician and the client are *test* situations. The clinician is continually testing the response of the client in terms of its correctness and the effects of her rewards and penalties on the frequency of occurrence of behaviors and the approach motivation and avoidance motivation of the client. This testing is vital since it, and it alone, determines if a transaction needs to be repeated or if the therapy can move ahead. The testing will give the clinician much insight into the cognitive level of the client. Testing also tells the clinician if she can continue working on the speech behavior or if she must work on the client's attending behavior. The testing determines what the response of the clinician will be to the client. And it is *imperative* that there be a response from the clinician, some sort of acknowledgment that at least indicates that the clinician was aware that the client responded. One way to extinguish a newly created behavior in therapy is to not respond to it. If there is no consequence for a behavior, there is no reason to perform the behavior. For example, students have approach motivation and study for examinations because there is a consequence, the reward of a good grade. Or could it be avoidance motivation, to avoid a failing grade? Now, if there is no consequence for a speech behavior, no response from the clinician, the client will have no approach motivation to achieve a reward or avoidance motivation to avoid a penalty.

Later in the clinical process we withdraw the reward, but this is for a very special reason we discuss in another chapter. For now, we view the response of the clinician to the client's behavior as a vital component in the clinical interaction between the clinician and the client. It is an essential part of the learning process, especially when the new behavior is just being introduced.

THE CLINICAL INTERACTION MODEL

The Clinical Interaction Model (CIM) is developed by combining various aspects of the learning theories and concepts with the clinician/client S — O — R/S — O — R transaction. In each transaction the clinician, as shown in Figure 4, has three clinical tasks she must perform if the transaction is to be completed. She must provide the initial stimulus, evaluate the client's response, and deliver her response. We will discuss each of these tasks.

Antecedent Events: The Clinician's Stimulus

Modeling. One of the ways we can make therapy more efficient is to present the client with the behavior change goal. We can show, or model, the behavior; demonstrating or modeling articulation sounds, forms of syntax, new voice quality, or fluency controls for the stutterer. Teaching through modeling is one of our most important teaching techniques and has been used by speech clinicians for many years. Remember, this is the way many speech clinicians learn the *how* of therapy. Think of those students who observed my therapy with Gary and what they learned.

Guidance. As was pointed out earlier, guidance is leading or directing the client to the correct behavior. The guidance may be verbal, gestural, environmental, or physical. We provide verbal guidance when we say to a client, "Can you make the sound just like I did?" or "How do we ask for water?" These are prompts to get the client to produce a behavior without modeling it. Gestural guidance includes those facial expressions and body or hand gestures we use to prompt a behavior; for example, if we have a client with a vocal pitch problem and we use a hand gesture to cue the client to raise or lower his pitch we are using gestural guidance. Environmental guidance occurs when we manipulate the stimuli in the client's surroundings in such a way that the desired behavior occurs. For example, if we were working on sucking behavior, we might prompt it by having a glass of juice with a straw in it sitting on a table in front of the client. An example of physical guidance would be the manipulation of the mouth as in the moto-kinesthetic method of articulation therapy.

Information. We can provide our clients with two types of information, *behavior* and *general* information. The behavioral information is used to supplement the model of the behavior. We can give the client instructions on how he should hold his mouth or on tongue placement. The information given here is directly related to the performance of the behavior we are teaching. General information occurs at any time during therapy and consists of any information that the clinician gives the client that is not directly related to the speech behavior. It includes, among other things, setting up future appointments or giving instruction on home programs.

Evaluation: The Clinician's Cognitions

The clinician has four important decisions to make before she can respond to the client. *First,* she must evaluate the correctness of the response. This determines whether she rewards the production or penalizes it. *Second,* she must determine if the correct response is occurring more often and the incorrect response is occurring less often. This tells her if her reward and penalty are functioning as they should or if she needs to change them. *Third,* she needs to evaluate the attentiveness of the client to the therapy. If the client is not attending, then she must reevaluate her reward and penalty since these are her tools to create approach motivation and avoidance motivation in the client. *Fourth,* she must determine how she will initiate the next transaction. This is dependent on the first three decisions she has made. She may move ahead with therapy if the client's response was correct or she may repeat the last transaction if the response was incorrect. Further, if the client is not attending to therapy, she may deal with the factor of attention through the client's approach or avoidance motivation.

In addition to making the four decisions discussed above, the clinician must also be aware of the client's attitudes, emotions, and feelings during the transactions. As long as these factors are not negatively influencing the treatment program, the clinician does no more than monitor them. But, if any of these factors begin to interfere with therapy, the clinician will have to deal with it. In fact, the basic therapy plan may have to be temporarily set aside while the clinician deals with, for example, the client's attitude. Dealing with the client's attitudes, emotions, and feelings is discussed in Chapter 8.

The response of the clinician to the client's behavior performance is an extremely important part of therapy. If the clinician's response is a reward, she is creating approach motivation in the client. He is motivated to get the reward and will attend to therapy and perform the appropriate speech behavior so he can get the reward. On the other hand, if her response is a penalty, she is creating avoidance motivation in the client. He is motivated to avoid the penalty and will attend to therapy and not perform the incorrect speech behavior that results in the penalty. Motivation, in one form or another, is essential for successful therapy.

These are powerful incentives that are under the control of the clinician. Careful planning and observations on the part of the clinician will make her reward responses effective for encouraging performance of the correct speech behavior and attending behavior. At the same time, her penalty responses will discourage incorrect speech performance and nonattending behavior. Conversely, nonattending behaviors will occur less often when they are penalized. We must keep in mind that, in therapy, we are concerned with two forms of behavior, that is, speech behavior and attending behavior.

Contingent Events: The Clinician's Response

Reward. As was mentioned earlier, reward is the same thing as reinforcement. It is an event that occurs after the behavior is performed and which the client views as a positive event. If the client feels that the contingent event is a reward, the probability that the behavior will occur again is increased. The client is highly motivated to get the reward and will perform the appropriate behavior to be rewarded. Approach motivation is important in therapy. There is a danger here, though. Many times clinicians decide that something will be rewarding to the client when it actually is not. We cannot determine if something is rewarding until we see the effect it has on the client's behavior. If we respond to a client in a certain way several times and the behavior we are responding to increases in frequency of occurrence, then, and only then, can we say that the response is rewarding. Remember, the reward is for the *client*, not you. You may like chocolate and enjoy eating it; however, if your client has an allergic reaction and breaks out in a rash, the chocolate is not rewarding to him. His only rewarding behavior is scratching. Obviously, we must predetermine what we are going to use as a reward and we base this decision on past clinical experience. We must also remember to observe the effect of our reward on the client to see if our decision was correct.

The importance of observing the effect of the reward on the behavior is clearly illustrated in a published report by a clinician. In this report, the clinician indicated that he "rewarded" stuttering behavior by having a female clinician kiss the stutterer each time he had a block. The occurrence of stuttering behavior all but disappeared and the clinician then concluded that stuttering behavior does not follow the operant principle of increase in frequency of occurrence with contingent reward. The clinician was observant and noted that the behavior changed in frequency of occurrence. But, he failed to realize that the kiss from the female clinician was functioning as a *penalty* rather than a reward. The clinician based his determination of a reward on his own values, but his guess was wrong. Even though "kiss therapy" appears to reduce stuttering, I would hesitate to recommend it. The treatment program might create a few problems for both you and your client.

There are two types of rewards we can give our clients. Primary rewards meet basic needs such as food and water. Secondary rewards have a more social impact and are learned, such as telling the child "good" after a production or patting him on the head. We must be concerned with both the strength of the reward and how appropriate it is for our clinical setting. If someone offered you $.50 to type a 10-page paper for him, you would probably turn down the offer.

But, if he offered you $500, you would rush to your typewriter. This is approach motivation. The strength of the reward is very important and is determined by the client. If there is good rapport between the client and the clinician the reward is strengthened since the clinician is an important person to the client. Furthermore, it is important to remember that what may be a powerful reward for you may not be for your client. The appropriateness of the reward is also very important. If the reward is a very chewy gum candy, therapy must wait until it is eaten, which might take a considerable amount of time. If we do use a consumable reward, we must decide when it is to be consumed, during therapy or after therapy.

We must also consider the timing of the reward. If there is a lengthy period of time between the performance of the behavior and the presentation of the reward, the association of the reward and the behavior may be lost. The client might have performed another behavior in the meantime and, since the reward is most contingent to this behavior, this is the one that is rewarded. For example, the client performs the appropriate speech behavior and follows this by scratching his nose. The clinician then gives the client the reward. The clinician is now rewarding the scratching which increases in frequency of occurrence. *Rewards should be given immediately after the desired behavior has been performed.*

Finally, we need to consider the schedule of presentation of the reward. If we reward each and every performance of the behavior, this is a *continuous reward schedule.* The ratio here is for every response there is a reward, a 1:1 ratio. As was discussed earlier, this leads to rapid learning. But, when the reward is removed, there is also rapid extinction; the behavior disappears quickly without the reward. We can also use an *intermittent reward schedule.* If we reward every third preformance of the behavior, we are using a *fixed ratio,* that is, a ratio of 3:1. The fixed ratio can be varied according to the response of the client.

It is very important we recognize that when we move from a 1:1 ratio (continuous reward) to a 2:1 ratio (intermittent reward) that we are actually going from a 100% reward schedule to a 50% reward schedule. This is quite a large step, too large for some clients. This step can be reduced if we adjust the ratio by adding zeros; for example, changing the 1:1 ratio to a 10:10 ratio. This is actually the same ratio but now we can manipulate it into smaller steps by moving to a 10:9 ratio. We are now rewarding 9 of 10 performances or a 90% schedule of reward. We can then adjust it downward to a 10:8 ratio, a 10:7 ratio, and so forth. These smaller steps of the withdrawal of the reward may be necessary for some of our clients.

We can also use a variable ratio. This means that we might reward the third, fifth, and ninth performances. There is no set number of performances that must occur between rewards. You might even reward several performances in a row and then skip one. Intermittent reward is not as efficient in terms of quick learning of a behavior but it does make the behavior extremely stable in terms of continued existence after the reward is removed. Behaviors learned under this schedule of reward are almost impossible to extinguish. Both continuous and intermittent schedules are important in the clinical process as we shall see in later chapters.

The fixed interval and variable interval schedules have limited use for the speech clinician. However, we can use this technique to work on the duration of a behavior. For example, we might use either the fixed or variable interval schedule to extend the time a child would remain in his chair. The rewards would extend the amount of time the child remained seated. We would control this by varying the amount of time between rewards.

We cannot leave the concept of reward without acknowledging that there are many people who object to this form of therapy. Their objection is to *bribing* clients to work on their speech. The word *bribe* certainly does have negative connotations. I prefer to view the reward as payment for work done. When I am confronted with the bribe concept, I ask the person if they are bribed where they work. The answer is always a firm "No." I then ask them if they would continue to work if their company or agency decided not to pay them their salary. Again, the answer is "No." Now I ask you, the reader, is the salary one receives for work done a reward or a bribe? When we reward a client for work done, it is not a bribe, it is a reward that the client has earned through his effort. Then, again, who really cares what the motive is for the client as long as he is learning to perform the desired behavior?

Penalty. As was mentioned earlier, when a behavior is penalized it tends to occur less often. We focus our therapy on the production of the correct behavior and we often tend to ignore incorrect productions. Extinction theory indicates that if a behavior has no contingent event, it will no longer occur. However, this is a slow process for the speech clinician. Many clinicians respond to incorrect productions by telling the client, "That was not very good, let's try it again." This is a penalty. Let us not think of penalty in terms of capital or corporal punishment. The clinician is providing feedback to the client that the production was not correct. This is a penalty and results in the decrease in occurrence of the incorrect behavior. The client has avoidance motivation to avoid the penalty and will not perform the behavior that results in the penalty. This is much more efficient than waiting for the incorrect response to extinguish over time. We must take the same precautions with a penalty that we took with the reward. We must determine if our response is truly a penalty, control the strength of the penalty, and be concerned with the appropriateness of the penalty. To determine if the response is a penalty, we must determine its effect on the behavior. We must also be careful not to apply too great a penalty. This can create problems with morale. And, of course, we must be careful not to use a penalty that is not appropriate to our clinical setting. Last, but not least, we must be consistent in applying the penalty.

There are two basic forms of penalty. We can administer a penalty, such as making the client pick up things he has thrown on the floor, or make him stop and repeat a sound if he has made it incorrectly. On the other hand, we can penalize a client by taking something positive away from him, such as removing a token when he makes the incorrect sound. If the client has earned 20 tokens to purchase a reward after therapy and we take one away, this is a penalty. Knowing that if he makes the incorrect production he will lose one token, the client will have avoidance motivation to avoid this by not making the incorrect production. To make this more meaningful, consider what your response would be if every time you were late for class or late for work, you lost five of our society's tokens ($5, since our monetary system is a token economy). I doubt if you would be late again. You would have avoidance motivation to escape this penalty.

As with the case of rewarding our clients, there are also many people who object to the concept of penalizing a client. In fact, there is a more negative reaction to penalty as a teaching tool than there is to reward. One can always be kind to another person but it is difficult to be unkind. People often confuse being unkind with administering a penalty. I find it very interesting that all parents use some form of penalty as they raise their children but they then object to the use of penalty in other learning environments. Sometimes we can be very unkind by *not* penalizing a child. We are not providing the child with a learning experience. When we stop to think about it, much of our learning was based on penalty and the avoidance of penalty. When I learned to ride a bicycle one of the strongest factors in learning to balance the bike was to avoid the cuts and bruises that were a part of falling. And who cannot remember spankings, either of hands or that part of the body that is the seat of most spankings? How do most children learn not to "sass" their parents? Penalty is a very important part of human learning. And, the form of penalty we are using in therapy is not physical in nature. We leave this to parents.

The Model

Now that we understand the basic concepts involved in our cognitive behavior therapy, it is time to present a diagram or "model" which shows the interrelationships of the concepts in a clinical sense. The Clinical Interaction Model (CIM) is presented in Figure 5. The form of the model is based on the individual clinical transaction as presented in Figure 4. The model also includes the strategies and procedures (both cognitive and behavioral) that the clinician uses. It is important to note that the CIM includes transactions directed to both the speech behaviors and attending behaviors. The clinician should attempt to focus therapy on the speech behaviors but, if there are attending problems, the model shows you how to deal with the problem behaviors and regain both the attending behaviors and motivation in one form or another. The model is now complete with all of the various procedures and techniques the clinician will use in her transactions. This model will serve as your guide in the planning of therapy, for all clinical transactions, and in solving problems when your therapy is not providing the results your desire.

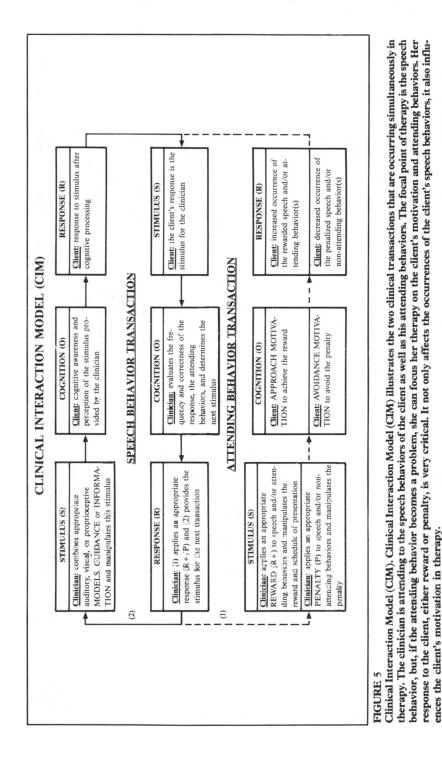

FIGURE 5

Clinical Interaction Model (CIM). Clinical Interaction Model (CIM) illustrates the two clinical transactions that are occurring simultaneously in therapy. The clinician is attending to the speech behaviors of the client as well as his attending behaviors. The focal point of therapy is the speech behavior, but, if the attending behavior becomes a problem, she can focus her therapy on the client's motivation and attending behaviors. Her response to the client, either reward or penalty, is very critical. It not only affects the occurrences of the client's speech behaviors, it also influences the client's motivation in therapy.

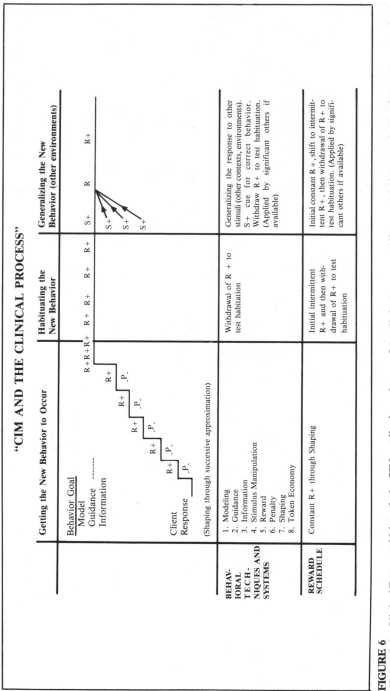

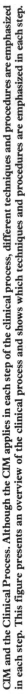

FIGURE 6

CIM and the Clinical Process. Although the CIM applies in each step of the clinical process, different techniques and procedures are emphasized in each step. This figure presents an overview of the clinical process and shows which techniques and procedures are emphasized in each step.

The CIM applies to all interactions with the client. However, it forms the core of therapy in the clinical process, the last three steps of a treatment program, that is, getting the new behavior to occur, habituating the new behavior, and generalizing the new behavior. To give you an overview of the clinical process and how the CIM relates to each phase of therapy, all factors are combined and shown in Figure 6. This figure is a guide for the rest of the book where we discuss each step in detail. It is a *map* of where we are going, not where we have been. It will take on added significance as we progress with our discussion and will eventually serve as a handy reference for you, providing you with an overview of your therapy. As you examine the figure you will note that the clinical techniques and procedures used by the clinician are listed under each step. For example, under the step "Getting the New Behavior to Occur," eight techniques and procedures are listed. These are the techniques and procedures that we use in our CIM for this step in the clinical process. However, let me remind you again that the CIM applies to all transactions we have with clients or significant others, be it in the evaluation, during conferences or counseling, or in direct therapy.

STIMULUS MANIPULATION WITH THE CIM

Stimulus Control

Antecedent events can be manipulated and used clinically in special ways. This is stimulus control which is important in all phases of the clinical process but especially in generalizing the new behavior. The client becomes conditioned to the various stimuli in his environment. These conditioned stimuli then play a very important and unique role in the client's learning experience.

Stimulus Roles

We have discussed the stimulus in the context of this book as anything in the environment that attracted the attention of the client and brought about a reaction. There are an unlimited number of stimuli in the client's environment but, for the sake of our discussion, we will limit ourselves to three general types of stimuli. First, there are the people in the client's environment. They include all of the people who interact with the client. We will also consider here what these people do, such as their verbal statements, their gestures, and their expressions. The people are the source of many stimuli. The next general type of stimuli are speaking situations the client experiences. These are special speaking situations which, particularly for the client who stutters, elicit an emotional response. These speaking situations include both specific ones like speaking before groups and general speaking environments such as at home or at school. The third type of stimuli are objects in the client's environment such as the tape recorder in the clinic room or, for the stutterer, the telephone. We will now extend the concept of these stimuli to include the special roles that they assume after they have been associated with a specific contingent event.

Conditioned Stimuli

When a stimulus is consistently associated with a reward or a penalty, the stimulus becomes conditioned. That is, the stimulus takes on a special characteristic or role, cuing the client as to what the outcome will be if a particular behavior is performed. These stimuli are known as discriminative stimuli. They do not elicit the response like a tap on the knee elicits a knee jerk. Rather, they provide the client with a *clue* as to what is going to happen if they perform the behavior associated with the stimulus. These cues have a definite influence on the probability of the behavior occurring. Let us consider some general examples of stimuli that have been conditioned and assumed special roles.

Positive stimuli. First of all, there are those stimuli which have been conditioned to a positive outcome, a reward. We refer to these conditioned stimuli as positive stimuli, or S+. A steak on a platter has become an S+ to most of us, signifying to us that if we sit down and eat the steak the outcome will be rewarding. This stimulus was not always a conditioned stimulus. It only assumed the role of an S+ after we had eaten and enjoyed the first steak and made the association between the steak and the reward of eating it. We will ignore the penalty of paying for the steak since this ruins the analogy. We also learned to answer the telephone in this way. The telephone ring means nothing to the very young child. But, when the telephone ringing is associated with answering the telephone and talking to someone we know, the reward changes the character of the telephone ringing.

Stimuli in the therapy environment quickly assume the role of S+ when rewards are presented. The clinician presents the rewards for specific behaviors. When the client sees the clinician, her presence cues him that if he performs the behavior he will be rewarded. Even the clinic room becomes associated with the reward and provides a cue for the correct behavior. This might tend to explain why most clinicians have had the experience of the client speaking extremely well in the therapy room and then reverting back to the old speech as soon as he leaves the clinical environment. We make great progress in the therapy room, but the parents report that he is making no progress in the home. When there is no S+ in his environment, there is no prompting for the correct speech behavior to occur.

Negative stimuli. Other stimuli become associated with a negative outcome, a penalty. We will refer to these conditioned stimuli as negative stimuli, or S-. An example of this would be our first experience with a "No Left Turn" sign where we received a traffic ticket. Either we had seen the sign and ignored it or we had seen it but it did not register with us. In any event, even though we pleaded our innocence with the traffic officer, told him that the sign was located in such a way that it could not be seen from where our car was located, insisted that the sign was covered with snow even though it was July, and other equally valid arguments, we received a traffic ticket. This cost us between $10 and $20. After paying the fine the sign took on significant meaning. We looked for "No Turn" signs and, indeed, did not turn. The sign cued us that if we did turn we would get a ticket and have to pay another fine. So we avoided the penalty of the fine by not performing the turn. We substituted another behavior, going straight ahead, and this allowed us to escape the penalty. There are innumerable examples of this type of learning in our lives where we avoid penalties by performing different behaviors.

Just as with the S+, the clinician quickly assumes the S- role in the clinic room. If the client knocks all of the materials off the clinic table onto the floor and the clinician then makes him pick up all of the materials, she is applying the penalty and becomes associated with it. When the client enters the room he is cued that if he knocks the things off the clinic table, he will be penalized. Therefore, he performs another behavior to avoid the penalty; he does not knock the things off the clinic table. This same avoidance behavior occurs when the clinician assigns some sort of penalty to the production of the incorrect speech behavior. She becomes an S- for the incorrect production, cuing that if it is produced it will be penalized. The client then attempts to avoid the penalty by performing some other behavior. If the clinician has already taught the correct behavior, this would be the client's choice since the correct behavior not only avoids the penalty but also achieves the reward.

Neutral stimuli. So far, the clinician plays two stimulus roles in the clinic room; S+, prompting the correct production of the speech behavior, and S-, prompting the avoidance of the penalty by not producing the incorrect behavior. However, there is a third role that the stimulus can assume. This is the neutral stimulus or S0. This stimulus signals the client that there will be no reward for the behavior. Since the behavior is not rewarding (or rewarded), there is no reason for the behavior to exist. Thus, it extinguishes, it no longer occurs since it serves no function. The contingent event in this instance is zero.

Stimulus Manipulation

All stimuli can be manipulated by the clinician. The manipulation can take several forms, such as changing the strength of the stimulus or shifting the role of the stimulus. This is a vitally important clinical procedure which we will use with the CIM in all phases of the clinical process. We will discuss each of the techniques involved in stimulus manipulation.

Shifting the role of the stimuli. Although a stimulus may have assumed the role of an S+, S-, or S0, these roles can be changed. If, for example, the parents have consistently penalized the client for his speech, their role is an S-. But if, through counseling, they no longer react to the client's speech, their role will shift to S0. If, on the other hand, the parents are rewarding the client's speech problem and maintaining it in the home environment, their role as S+

can be changed to that of S0 by removing the reward. The role of the stimulus can, therefore, be changed by associating the stimulus with a different conting-ent event. This becomes very important as we attempt to generalize the new speech behaviors into other environments. We can utilize the stimulus roles of the significant others in these environments to cue the new speech behaviors to occur in their presence. This is the key to carry-over. The following illustration indicates that role shift is accomplished by associating the stimulus with a new contingent event. If the parents were only associated with penalty for behavior, their role is S–. But if the parents are then associated with reward for the behavior, their role shifts to S+.

To Shift		Change Contingent Event	
From / To		From / To	
S–, S0 / S+		P, 0 / R+	
S+, S0 / S–		R+, 0 / P	
S+, S– / S0		R+, P / 0	

Gradual introduction to stimuli. As we generalize a new bahavior into other speaking environments, we may find that a certain stimuli is an S– and too threatening for the client. We then have to present the stimulus gradually as the client adjusts to it. For example, a client who stutters might have great fear associated with speaking in front of groups (S–). For this client we gradually introduce the speaking situation. We do this by starting with one listener where the client can perform satisfactorily (S+). We then add another listener. This process is repeated so that we are gradually introducing the stimuli while keeping the talking situation at a level where the client can deal with it. We can gradually increase the frequency of the stimuli, the strength or intensity of the stimuli, or the duration of the stimuli. The procedure is as follows:

$$_{s+} — R — R+$$
$$_{s+} — R — R+$$
$$S+ — R — R+$$
$$S+ — R — R+$$

Gradual withdrawal of stimuli. This is also knows as *fading.* We gradually withdraw the stimulus by presenting it less often, in a less complete form, or for a shorter period of time. We fade the speech model as the new speech behavior is learned. This helps make the behavior independent of the model. As was mentioned earlier, we can manipulate the frequency, intensity, or duration of the stimuli. Remember that the completeness of the stimuli is involved here. This form of manipulation is seen below.

$$S+ \; - \; R \; - \; R+$$
$$S+ \; - \; R \; - \; R+$$
$$s+ \; - \; R \; - \; R+$$
$$s+ \; - \; R \; - \; R+$$
$$R \; - \; R+$$

Increase the number of stimuli. The clinician might also have to increase the number of stimuli in the client's environment. These stimuli (S+) would then cue the new speech behavior to occur in other environments. She must create more S+ in the client's nonclinical environment so the new speech behaviors are cued to occur in the home, at school, and on the job. This manipulation system can be illustrated as follows:

S+———R———R+   S+ = Clinical environment
(S+)   S+ = Home environment
(S+)   S+ = School environment

Decrease the number of stimuli. The clinician can exert some control over the number of stimuli in the client's clinical environment. If the client is overwhelmed by the number of stimuli and distracted from therapy, the clinician can remove or mask stimuli that might distract the client.

Some objects can be physically removed from the clinic room such as toys and clinical materials not to be used in the particular therapy session. Other things, such as a wall-mounted mirror, cannot be removed; but they can be covered, or seating arranged in such a way as to reduce their influence. Let us view this means of stimulus manipulation in this way:

$$S+ \; - \; R \; - \; R+$$
$$\cancel{S+} \; - \; \cancel{R} \; - \; \cancel{R+}$$
$$\cancel{S+} \; - \; \cancel{R} \; - \; \cancel{R+}$$

RESPONSE MANIPULATION WITH THE CIM

Shaping

Shaping is an operant technique used to create a new behavior, a behavior that the client cannot perform. In shaping, the goal behavior is *not* set forth for the client. This will be added later, but is not part of *pure* shaping. When shaping is used, any behavior that occurs which the clinician feels approximates the goal behavior, determined by the clinician, is rewarded. The principle here is that the reward will increase the likelihood that this behavior will occur again. At the same time, behaviors that do not approximate the goal receive no contingency. This means that those behaviors will extinguish because there is no reward. The process is referred to as *successive approximation*. The technique was developed in work with animals in experimental laboratories. There is no cognition involved in the process. If the speech clinician uses this technique in its pure form it is very inefficient. The client does not know what the goal behavior is and the occurrences of approximated behaviors occur randomly.

Token Economy

The token economy is a very special system of providing rewards for a client. One of the problems with giving specific rewards is that clients tend to tire of being give the same reward over a period of time. There is also the problem of finding a single reward that is meaningful to a group of clients. The token economy solves these two problems. The tokens are saved by the clients to purchase rewards after therapy or at a specific time that will not interfere with therapy. The token can be anything that the clinician has at hand; pieces of paper, poker chips, or checkers. They are given to the client in the place of a specific reward. The tokens themselves become rewarding after the client has actually purchased one of the backup rewards. This reward system allows the clinician to select a number of rewards, with different "prices," so that the client has a choice of what kind of reward he prefers. The number of tokens given in the clinical situation is determined by the clinician as is the "price" of each item the client can purchase. The clinician will adjust this as she finds herself spending too much of her money on rewards. As with our own economy, inflation will set in and the prices of the rewards will increase.

Eventually, all token economies must come to an end. The rewards must be withdrawn as the behavior becomes more firmly established. The token reward should be paired with verbal praise during the token economy. The tokens can then be withdrawn as the verbal praise is maintained. This reduces the influence of the backup reward as the behavior is becoming stable.

The token economy has many advantages over a traditional reward program. Some advantages are providing a variety of rewards, not interrupting therapy while the client consumes a reward, making it easier for the clinician to administer the initial reward, and administering the same initial reward to all of the clients in a group setting. Tokens are very powerful rewards and the token economy a powerful teaching/learning tool. Consider what would happen if you were given $1 for each minute you were early for work or for class.

What about a token economy with older clients? I have used a token economy with clients of all ages. With a 17-year-old client who stuttered, I arranged a token economy in the home where he received a token for controlled fluent speech but lost two tokens each time he talked without his controls. What was his reward? When he collected a certain number of tokens he could use the family car for a date. Another client, 37 years of age, had two cars. One was a large family station wagon and the other a foreign sports car. The token economy was set up where his wife would give tokens for the correct behavior and take them away for the incorrect behavior. The tokens were counted each morning and the number of tokens determined if the client drove the sports car to work or had to drive the station wagon. The client had a lot of avoidance motivation to avoid having to take the station wagon to work. It takes a little imagination and a great deal of cooperation to use the token economy with older clients but, if it can be arranged, it is well worth the time and effort. Finally, did the client with the two cars divorce his wife because he had to drive the station wagon? No, he sold it and bought a second sports car. You have to be on your toes to keep ahead of your clients.

CLIENT MOTIVATION AND THE CIM

Can we assume that all of our clients are interested in working on their communication problems? Absolutely not. We might think of dividing clients into two groups, children and adults, but this is not the case. Perhaps a more plausible division might be based on why they came to us in the first place. Clients come to us either because they want help and are searching it out, or because some other person in their environment has made the decision for them. This is not a foolproof system but it is the best that I have been able to come up with. Let us pursue it a bit further. If a client himself wants help with his communication problem, I can assume that there is a degree of approach motivation that I can work with. I can also increase this approach motivation through my reward system in the clinical environment.

But what about the client who is sent to us for therapy? It is not the client's choice to come to us; he is forced to attend therapy. What do we do here? We must attempt to create "artificial" approach motivation in the clinical environment through our reward system. If we are clever enough, this will suffice in this environment, but we will have to make further adjustments when we try to generalize the behavior to other environments where we do not have direct control over the reward system. Let us take each of these conditions, motivated clients and unmotivated clients, and discuss the clinical ramifications of their attitude toward therapy.

Clients Seeking Therapy

We can make an assumption that clients who come to us seeking assistance have some interest in therapy. Although we are not faced with creating approach motivation in these clients, we still must maintain it. We can accomplish this through our reward system. However, there is a point in many treatment programs where the client loses his approach motivation. As we get closer to the end of therapy and the new speech behavior is almost perfect, approach motivation wanes. If we cannot find an appropriate reward that will maintain the needed approach motivation, perhaps we can find a penalty which the client wants to avoid. We can then use the client's avoidance motivation as a means of maintaining interest in the therapy.

We can also turn to the significant others in the client's external environment to help us maintain approach motivation and avoidance motivation. But, we cannot always count on the assistance of significant others. We have two alternatives regarding their participation, which we will discuss here briefly and then in more detail in later chapters.

Cooperative significant others. When we are lucky enough to have significant others who will become involved and assist our client, we can use them in several ways. The most important way we can use them is to create a support system: that is, to make sure that the significant others understand what the client is working on and provide him with moral support as he is resolving his communication problem. It is nice to be appreciated and it is also nice to have others acknowledge and reward our effort. The significant others must be counseled to reward the client's efforts and support him through understanding and, perhaps, even direct assistance. With cooperation from the significant others we will be able not only to get the new behavior to occur more rapidly, but we will also be able to generalize the new behavior faster.

Uncooperative or absent significant others. The task of maintaining the approach motivation of the client is a more difficult task when the only people involved in maintaining motivation are the clinician and the client. Essentially, the client has no support system. We might be able to compensate for this in some way, such as bringing teachers, nurses, and other people involved with the client into the picture even though they are not truly significant to the client. Again, if we can get these people to provide moral support and understanding, the task is easier. The rewards provided by these people are very important as a supplement to the direct therapeutic rewards that we are providing. We have a real challenge here but it is imperative that we maintain the client's interest in therapy. Can we also use avoidance motivation with these surrogate significant others? Yes, but this must be done with caution. They are not sophisticated clinicians. They will need close supervision in the application of penalty, but, if the penalty is administered properly, the client's avoidance motivation will be an important factor. The main problems we face when using a variety of people as a support system are consistency and coordination of their efforts.

Clients Sent for Therapy

The type of client who is sent for therapy is not limited to children whose parents or teachers feel that therapy is needed. He could also be an adult aphasic, adult stutterer, or any other type of client who, himself, does not really see the need for therapy. In some instances, a business will recommend therapy for an employee if they feel that he does not have the communication skills that they deem necessary. In any event, both children and adults are included in this category of clients who really do not have an interest in working on their speech. With this type of client we really have a problem. We must create approach motivation if our treatment is going to be effective. Our alternatives are very limited here. We will probably not have much success trying to create interest by talking to the client, especially with a younger client. This does not mean that we should not try approaching the client on a cognitive level. It simply means that we need to supplement our cognitive interaction with a reward program that will create approach motivation. Artificial though it may be, if we can create approach motivation to get the reward, we have accomplished our goal of getting the person to learn the new speech behavior. As we said earlier, as long as the client is learning the new behavior, the reasons he is learning are not important.

For both the client who enters therapy with a high degree of interest and the sent clients, the approach motivation may wane as we progress in therapy. Again, we may have to create avoidance motivation in the client and use this to maintain interest. We can also use the help of the significant others if they are available.

Cooperative significant others. With clients sent for therapy we need a strong support system and we are fortunate to have cooperative significant others. The client needs all of the support and understanding that the others in his life can give him. A meaningful reward program is vitally important in the external environment, especially when we attempt to generalize the new behavior to that environment. The clinician must do some very careful counseling with the significant others so that they not only understand that lack of interest on the part of the client, but also how their support and reward system will help the client in therapy. Careful supervison of this support system is vital. The supervision can be in the form of reports, but, in one way or another, the clinician must be aware of what is transpiring in the external environment.

Uncooperative or absent significant others. If we have any clinical expertise, we need it most when we are faced with a client who has no desire to be in therapy and no one in the client's environment is there for support. We can create approach motivation in the clinic room but the minute the client leaves this environment, there is no support or encouragement from significant others. The best we can do is to enlist the help of other people in the client's environment (teachers, nurses, occupational therapists, physical therapists, physicians, etc.) and make the most of the support that they will give us in providing external rewards for the client. All is not lost in this situation but our clinical skills will be taxed to the utmost. The use of avoidance motivation through penalty can still be used in this situation but *extreme* caution must be used since the other people assisting us in providing penalty are not trained in our specialty. We are still faced with the problems of consistency and coordination of the efforts of people who agree to help us.

Chapter 3

Synopsis

We may now understand the role of the Clinical Interaction Model in therapy but, without the client's attention, the CIM is not operational. We can assist the client in focusing and maintaining his attention by creating a clinical environment which is conducive to learning. This *learning environment* is fundamental to any successful therapy program. With some exceptions, the clinician has control over the clinical environment and can modify it if it is interfering with therapy. This chapter deals with these issues as they relate to therapy.

Chapter 3

The Learning Environment

ATTENDING BEHAVIORS

The most important ingredient for learning is attention. If a student is not attending to lectures in classes, more than likely he is not learning anything. Of course there are professors where, even if you attend to their lectures, you do not learn anything. But let us hope that this is the exception rather than the rule. The same principle of attention applies to clients in therapy. If they are not attending to the therapy, they are not going to learn anything from the experience. The clinical process will not work if the client is not attending to therapy. There is an old story that tells about the importance of attention. It goes this way:

> A farmer once had a mule that knew how to do tricks. It was a highly trained mule and the farmer delighted in the fact that he had the only "educated" mule in the county. However, his crops failed one year and he desperately needed money to pay his debts on his farm. So, he had to face the prospect of selling his mule. Another farmer had heard about the "educated" mule and made the owner an offer he could not refuse. So, the new owner took the mule to his farm, called in his friends to see the mule's tricks, and proceeded to give the mule the commands to perform his various tricks. THE MULE JUST STOOD THERE! He did not do any of his tricks and all of the new owner's friends had a good laugh about how he had been fooled into thinking the mule could perform tricks. The very angry new owner took the mule back to the original owner and confronted him with the fact that the mule would not perform tricks. The original owner asked the new owner to show him how he went about getting the mule to perform. So, the new owner stood in front of the mule and gave all of the commands for the tricks. Again, the mule just stood there. The original owner's face lit up and he said, "No wonder he won't perform his tricks. You are doing it wrong." With that, the original owner went over to the wood pile and got a 2×4 about five feet long. He walked over in

front of the mule, and with a hefty swing, he broke it over the mule's head. Then he turned to the new owner and said, "First of all, you have to get his attention."

The moral of the story is that you must get the attention of your client before he will learn anything in your therapy. This is the first priority. So, you must create an environment in your clinic room that is conducive to learning, that is, an environment where the client will attend to you and your therapy rather than attend to some other stimuli in the environment.

SENSORY INTEGRATION

Human beings have basically five sensory channels for receiving stimuli. We can hear things through the auditory channel, see things through the visual channel, smell things through the olfactory channel, taste things through the gustatory channel, and feel things through the bodily sense channel. I have taken a few liberties with this last channel by combining factors such as kinesthesia, proprioception, and other body senses into a single channel for the sake of clarity. Be aware that this channel receives body sensory information from many sources.

We are under constant bombardment from a multitude of stimuli which we integrate into a meaningful unit, such that we can deal with in terms of adjustment to our environment. Important stimuli are attended to while unimportant stimuli are evaluated and then ignored. Take just a minute and try and figure out how many stimuli are impinging on you as you read this chapter. Consider the stimuli in your external environment that are attempting to get your attention. If you are in a library, where I have found it impossible to study, you find that there are people walking past you, there is the scraping of chairs as someone gets up from a study table, if the air conditioning or the heating is not working properly you may be either too cold or too hot, or your chair may not be comfortable. Regardless of where you are, stop reading for a moment and consider the number of potentially distracting stimuli there are in your environment, but do not get so distracted that you forget to come back to our discussion.

Now that your are back reading, let us consider the things that are going on inside of you, your internal environment, that are acting as stimuli, trying to get your attention. Your ears may still be ringing from the rock concert you went to last night, your head may ache from a cold, your stomach may be upset, your nose may be running from an allergy, or your eyes may hurt from too much reading (a common but unfounded complaint from many of my students). Again, stop reading for a moment and take an inventory of your internal stimuli. If you have all of the examples presented above, do not resume your reading. You are not really learning anything anyway since you are being distracted by all of these stimuli. Come back to the book when you are feeling better.

Finally, we add to the list internal thoughts, emotions, and feelings, which are also vying for your attention. How do we cope with all of these factors? How do we attend to any one thing? Humans have the ability to sort out the important stimuli and attend to these while the other stimuli are placed in the background. Even though we may be attending to one stimulus, if another stimulus is urgent, we will shift our attention to it. You are attending to your reading at this instance, but if you suddenly had a muscle cramp in your leg, your attention would shift to the pain in your leg. Once the pain left, you could shift back to reading.

THE FIGURE/GROUND CONCEPT

Figure/ground is a fundamental concept in Gestalt psychology. We have all seen examples of it in basic texts in psychology where an illustration shows a white vase against a black background or field. But, as we look at it, we suddenly see the profiles of two faces looking at each other. Now the profiles are black and the background or field is white. What we see depends on what we are attending to. This example concerns only the visual channel, but the same concept applies to all of the sensory channels in the human. How many times have you sat in a less-than-stimulating lecture and found yourself listening to noises out in the hall? Your auditory figure/ground shifted so that the noises were the figure while the lecture was the ground, or, instead of watching the professor draw diagrams on the board, you found yourself looking at the bald spot on his head. These examples illustrate a figure/ground problem within a particular sensory channel.

We can now extend this to figure/ground problems *between* channels. Let us go back to the boring lecture. We would both agree that the auditory channel should be the figure with all other channels being ground. However, the lecture is just before lunch and you missed breakfast that day. You now find that all of your attention is on how hungry you are and the lecture is background. Another example would be attempting to study when the television is on. The textbook is very stuffy and you find yourself listening to the soap opera. We have another figure/ground problem, but now we have channels shifting roles.

CLINICAL IMPLICATIONS

Could the figure/ground relationship possibly influence the transactions between the clinician and the client? Yes: If your client is attending to something other than you and your therapy, you will accomplish very little. Like the mule, first you must get the client's attention. This means that you, the clinician, must be the figure in the clinic room and determine which of the sensory channels you are going to use in your teaching. If you are going to produce the sound for the child to imitate, the figure channel you are using is the auditory channel. The visual channel may contribute some information, but the auditory channel is the primary source of information. On the other hand, if you are going to show the client where to place the tongue during the production, the visual channel is the primary source of information.

Your *first* clinical task is to determine which channel is going to be the figure channel. This will depend on what your clinical task is at the time. Your *second* task is to determine what the figure will be in the figure channel. Let us consider an example. You decide that the auditory channel is going to be the figure channel. Your task then is to make certain that the other channels are controlled to the extent that they will not interfere with your choice, they do not distract your client. You need to determine if there are visual, olfactory, or body sense stimuli in the clinic room that might interfere. We are not concerning ourselves with the gustatory channel since it is not a factor in this example. There always seems to be a mirror in a therapy room so you might seat the client in such a way that the reflection in the mirror is not distracting. The seating arrangement could also control the client's being distracted by a window in the room. If the room is extremely stuffy, you might open the door for a while and air out the room before therapy starts. Should the room have a shelf of toys that might distract the client, you could cover them with a cloth during therapy. When you control these potentially distracting stimuli, you are creating a learning environment. You are helping the client maintain his attention on you and your therapy.

Once you have the auditory channel as the figure channel, you must determine if there are other auditory stimuli which will interfere with the auditory figure/ground relationship. A clinician might have controlled all of the stimuli in the room that would cause a shift to another figure channel but still have a problem maintaining the figure/ground relationship within the figure channel she selected. Clinic rooms in the public schools have often been rooms that no one else needed or wanted. They are sometimes located right next to the bathrooms and every time a toilet is flushed, so is therapy. Who can resist listening to a toilet flush? Then there is the noise in the hallway. Is outside noise an insurmountable problem? Perhaps, in some instances, but if interfering sounds cannot be eliminated, they can sometimes be masked by a controlled sound in the clinic room. Once, when working in a clinic room where there was a great deal of distracting noise, I brought a portable radio into the room and tuned it to a local station that played nothing but soft, innocuous music, much like "Musak." I turned up the radio to the point that the music masked most of the extraneous noise and found that the client maintained his attention better during therapy. Yes, there are problems in creating and maintaining a learning environment for our clients, but we have already discussed the fact that the clinician should be cognitively involved in the therapy.

Finally, we have the presence of the clinician herself in the clinic room. We will deal with the clinician as a separate entity rather than as a part of the general environment in the clinic room. The clinician can create many problems herself in terms of disturbing the client's figure/ground relationships. Over many years of supervision I have witnessed some interesting problems in this vein.

One clinician, attempting to work in the auditory channel, could not get the client to maintain the figure/ground relationship. The client continued to shift to the visual channel. The clinician was wearing earrings that consisted of three successively smaller hoops suspended one within the other. The hoops rotated independently as the earrings themselves swung with each head movement. It was fascinating to watch, not only for the client but also for the supervisor. This might be appropriate for hypnosis, but not speech therapy. Jewelry can be very distracting, particularly for young clients with neurological involvement where there is already a problem of distractability. The clinician must take care to not provide distractions in dress, mannerisms, and other behaviors. They are self-defeating.

This concept of figure/ground relationships in the clinic room is shown in Figure 7. It should be carefully noted in this model that the client provides constant feedback to the clinician in terms of what he is attending to. The clinician must be attending to the client for this feedback to be of any value. This is part of the monitoring and evaluation that the clinician must do in each succeeding clinical transaction. With my client, Gary, I was too involved in attempting to follow my lesson plan to notice that Gary was not paying attention to me. This information was being provided for me but I was not attending to it. Therefore, I did not make the necessary changes to correct the problem.

Figure 7 also shows that the clinician has control over the external environment, that is, the clinic room. She can eliminate visually distracting items from sight by either removing them or masking them. She can also control the seating arrangement to control potentially distracting visual stimuli. Unfortunately, the clinician does not have direct control over the internal environment of the client. If the client is feeling ill, or has a headache, this will interfere with therapy by distracting the client. It may be best to terminate the therapy while the client is not feeling well since little, if anything, is going to be accomplished. However, this decision is dependent on the policy of the agency where the therapy is being provided.

The most pertinent example of the implementation of the figure/ground concept in therapy occurred in an agency where, as a clinician, I worked with children who had severe neurological problems. We did therapy with the children in a darkened, sound-treated room with the child placed in a bathtub filled with warm water. The only light in the room was a small flashlight which was directed at the face of the clinician. In some instances, the clinician would apply bright red lipstick to further call the child's attention to the mouth. When these children were freed of distracting stimuli and were able to concentrate on their clinical tasks, their performance improved dramatically. This was the ultimate in stimulus control. Recognizing that this was an artificial environment, as soon as the children were adjusted to this environment and performing their clinical tasks at a high level of proficiency, other stimuli were gradually introduced, being careful to present the stimuli at levels below the child's

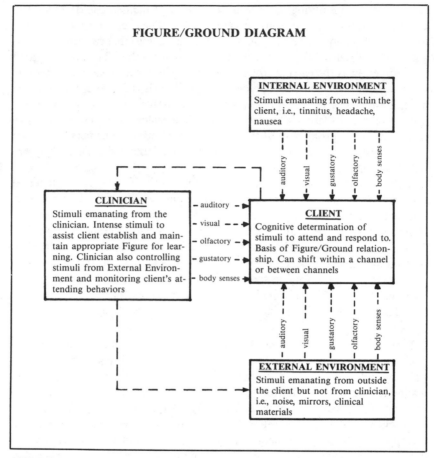

FIGURE 7
**Figure/Ground Diagram. The client receives stimuli through five sensory channels.
These stimuli emanate from three sources: his internal environment, his external
environment, and the clinician. The client determines which of the numerous stimuli to
attend to. This stimulus then becomes the figure while all remaining stimuli become
ground. The clinician must compete with other stimuli in order to get the client to
attend to therapy. Therapy then becomes the figure and all other stimuli are ground.**

threshold of distractability. Over a period of time, the children were able to work in a regular clinic room, maintaining their attention on therapy and not being distracted by the various stimuli in the room.

If the above example illustrated good utilization of the figure/ground control, let me give you another example and have you analyze it and see what is wrong with the clinical environment. The client in this example is a 16-year-old male with a slight voice quality disorder. The clinic room has a mirror along one wall, a chalk board on the opposite wall, and a large window on the outside wall. The clinician has arranged the table in the room so that when she is seated for therapy, her back is to the window and the client is facing her across the table. In order to brighten up the rather drab office, she has hung travel posters from Hawaii showing surfing and beach scenes on either side of the mirror and the chalk board. She has also hung along the top of the chalk board pictures her younger clients have drawn. The furniture in the room is for younger clients, and the only adult-sized chair she has is the one she uses. She has worn a heavy wool suit to work that day and, being warm, she opens the window a bit even though it is in the middle of winter. She keeps all of her clinical materials on the table in the room, including the stimulus cards for younger clients as well as toys, pencils, papers, and records.

When she dressed for work that day she decided to wear the wool suit and gold accessories. She put an intricate pin on the lapel of the suit, put on a gold charm bracelet and dangling earrings. She finished this off with three large gold rings, two on her right hand. She did her fingernails that day with a very bright red polish in order to set off the gold rings. The glasses she decided to wear had rhinestones in the frames, and she had her initials engraved in the lower lefthand corner of the left lens. The last thing she did before leaving for work was to splash on a generous dose of perfume.

I am sure that if you carefully study this example, you might find a few things that could interfere with the therapy interaction. This is, perhaps, an outlandish example, but how many of these things have you seen occurring in therapy you have observed? We are applying the "OP Rule" (other people) again.

We have gone from one extreme to another in terms of the clinical environment, but before we leave this topic we should deal with some practical problems in the clinic room. Let me give you an example of one such problem. The clinician I was observing was working with a 4-year-old child. The clinic room was furnished with two adult-sized chairs, two small chairs for children, and a table to hold the clinical materials. The therapy started with both the clinician and the child seated in the smaller chairs. Therapy was progressing nicely and the child was attending to all of the clinical activities. However, the clinician had some difficulty working with the materials on the table since she was sitting so low. She was also a bit uncomfortable sitting on such a small chair. She solved the problems by moving to an adult chair while the child remained in the small chair. The clinician could now use the materials on the table more easily and she was comfortable in the larger chair. This arrangement soon created other problems. The clinician now had to look down on the child since she was sitting so much higher. Further, since it was now easier to use the materials on the table, she made extensive use of them but the child was sitting so low he had trouble seeing what was happening. There was an obvious answer to all of this; place the child in an adult chair. This again placed the clinician and the child at about the same height and the child was now able to see the materials on the table. Things went fine for about 3 minutes and then the clinician began to lose the child's attention. He began to wiggle in the chair, swing his feet back and forth, and behave in a very restless fashion. The clinician tried to get his attention back on the therapy by increasing the rewards but was not successful. The remainder of the therapy session was not at all productive. The clinician was baffled since this was not typical behavior for this child.

During our conference on the therapy session I pointed out two possible explanations for this behavior. The most plausible explanation had to do with sitting in a chair where the feet do not touch the floor. This is very uncomfortable and the legs have a tendency to "go to sleep." The child's figure/ground relationship had shifted from attending to therapy to attending to the discomfort in his legs. He was wiggling and swinging his legs in order to prevent gangrene from setting in. If someone in the therapy session had to be uncomfortable, it should have been the clinician. She should be creating a comfortable learning environment for the child, not her.

There is still another possible explanation for this behavior in this child. This type of behavior is often seen in children who need to go to the toilet. Younger children may not ask if they can go to the toilet. They just wiggle more and more. They are obviously attending more to their bodily need than to therapy. More than one clinician has ignored these behavioral signs of impending disaster and had to clean up the clinic room. If in doubt, just ask. An ounce of prevention is worth a pound of paper toweling.

We mentioned clinical materials in earlier examples, but now let us be a bit more specific. Many speech clinicians going to a therapy session resemble a "bag lady." If you are not familiar with the term, it is used to describe women who carry all of their earthly possessions with them in a shopping bag. The therapist takes her bag of materials into the clinic room and proceeds to lay out all of the materials for the session on the table. She must have a game, a toy, or an instrument for every moment of therapy. There is no imagination evident in the therapy planning, just dependence on "gimmicks." The last thing the therapist takes out of the bag is a tape recorder so that she can record her therapy session (I wonder if these clinicians ever listen to their therapy). The table is now all but covered with games, books, pictures, toys, and the tape recorder. The clinician then brings the child into the clinic room and wonders why the child is not attending to therapy. The materials should have been left in the bag and the bag kept under the table. The tape recorder, if actually necessary, should be placed out of the child's direct line of vision, perhaps at the far end of the table. It might also be covered with a piece of cloth to mask it. There is nothing more distracting than clutter in a clinic room. Whatever happened to the speech clinician who could go into therapy with nothing more than a pencil and paper and motivate her clients?

Then there are mirrors. Every clinic room must have a mirror. The really good ones take up an entire wall. These large mirrors give the child twice as much to look at. And the clinician usually has the seating arranged in such a way that the mirror is either directly in front of the child or to one side of him. They may not be using the mirror as part of therapy, but the mirror is still there. Would it not make more sense to arrange the seating so that the mirror was not in the child's line of vision, perhaps with the mirror behind the child? If the mirror is needed for a segment of therapy, it is simply a matter of turning a chair around.

Mirrors take on added horror when they are "one-way" mirrors. These mirrors work fine until someone turns on a light in the observation room. You now have a "window" between the rooms. When the child sees other people watching him and then the light goes out and the "window" is a mirror again, you have a very distracted child. In one instance where this occurred the child had to be moved to another clinic room where there was no mirror, and finding one is no mean task. When the child saw the fleeting images of people in the mirror when the light was turned on briefly, he thought they were ghosts and that was the end of therapy in that room.

If you are working with a highly distractable child you should attempt to reduce the stimuli in your room as described earlier. You can also arrange the seating in such a way that the distractions in the room are minimized. You can place your chair in a corner of the room where there are no distracting stimuli behind you and place the child's chair facing you. In this way, the child has nothing to look at but you. This is a simple but effective way to control the child's attention.

One of the most ingenious devices you can use to work with a highly distractable client is the *pinhole mask*. This is simply a mask which you place over the client's eyes where he can only see out of two small pinholes. This serves to reduce the scope of the visual field. I saw this demonstrated with some severely involved cerebral palsied children and the effect it had on their coordination was startling. A severely involved athetoid who could barely walk due to head movements triggered by various stimuli in his visual field walked almost normally when wearing such a mask. With another client whose head movements triggered a series of reflexes which resulted in his falling out of his wheelchair, the pinhole mask eliminated the reflex chain and made it possible for him to receive therapy.

Before we leave the topic we must consider the effect that group therapy will have on the learning environment. As we add clients to the clinical environment, we are adding potentially distracting stimuli. This is an extremely important factor that we must consider when setting up group therapy. Some of our clients, because of age, maturity, type of disorder, or some other factor, may not be able to tolerate this increase in stimuli. There are no hard and fast rules to apply here. This is a clinical judgment that the speech clinician must make. She may decide that a certain client can tolerate the group setting but then find that the client cannot learn in such a setting. She may be able to modify the group setting in such a way that the client can operate satisfactorily but, if not, she will have to make some arrangements to provide the client with individual attention. The group therapy process is discussed in detail in Chapter 7.

Your challenge, as a speech clinician, is to create and maintain a clinical environment that is conducive to learning. Give your clients some assistance in maintaining their attention to your therapy. Make your therapy interesting. Show some enthusiasm. People pay attention to things that are interesting and entertaining. Therapy does not have to be a bore. The only person who can make therapy boring is the clinician. Is it unprofessional for the client to have fun in therapy, to enjoy therapy? Let us keep in mind that "awful" therapy creates many problems in figure/ground relationships. The client is confused. He often does not know which channel to attend to. And when he does know and attempts to attend to the figure channel, it is so boring and confusing he begins to attend to other channels. Think of your therapy as a television program and your client as the one who controls the dial on his television set. If your program is the best available, he will tune you in. However, if there is something better on another channel, he will tune to it and you have lost him. I have seen some therapy where I would have certainly understood if the client tuned his set to commercials since they were more interesting.

THE "HOW" OF THERAPY

Chapter 4

Synopsis

As we start our therapy, we concentrate on getting a new behavior to occur. The evaluation has been completed and we have decided on what our behavior change goal is. Our therapy plan has been formed and factors which might interfere with our therapy, such as a hearing loss or dysarthria, have been accounted for. We are now ready to introduce our client to the new behavior we plan to teach. This chapter discusses how the CIM is involved in getting the new behavior to occur.

Chapter 4

Getting the New Behavior to Occur

ANTECEDENT AND CONTINGENT EVENTS IN THE CIM

The focus in this phase of the clinical process is on the contingent events, the reward (R+) and penalty (P). We will use these contingent events to provide approach motivation and avoidance motivation for our clients. The consequences for the attempts by the client to produce the new speech behavior can both encourage the new behavior to occur, R+, or discourage the production of the original error, P. Remember that P is very important because the client succeeds in avoiding the penalty by performing the correct behavior. This is a very strong form of reward for the correct behavior. This is not to say that antecedent events are not important. We provide modeling, guidance, and information for the client, all of which are antecedent to the client's attempt to produce the new behavior. We then fade these events as the new behavior is learned.

We must also consider those clients where the behavior we are working with is not a totally *new* behavior. Perhaps we are working with a client who can produce the [g] in the initial position in a word but distorts it in all other positions. In this case we should view the *new* behavior not as the production of the [g] sound itself, but as the production of the correct [g] in medial and final positions of words. Fluency is not a *new* behavior for the stutterer. There are many times when the stutterer is completely fluent. We must get the client to the point where he can create fluent speech when he needs it in difficult speaking situations.

It is this phase of the clinical process that our clients are faced with their first major learning task. This is where they are going to "learn how to learn." We are emphasizing the contingent events because they provide the basis of learning, that is, attending to therapy as well as approach motivation and avoidance motivation to be an active participant in the clinical process. We will be using all of the techniques and procedures we discussed in Chapter 2 but we will combine them into an effective and efficient clinical approach.

COMBINING TECHNIQUES AND PROCEDURES

As we begin to combine the teaching techniques and procedures discussed in Chapter 2, we will gradually develop a more efficient and effective clinical approach. We start our therapy with the shaping procedure. A clinical example will help illustrate this point. We then add other techniques and processes, discussing how each addition has influenced therapy with a specific client.

Shaping

The speech clinician has determined that the client has a defective [s] sound. She talks with the client and when an [s] sound occurs that more closely approximates the correct production, she rewards it. She does not tell the client why he is receiving the reward, it is just given. This is shaping in its purest form. However, this type of clinical activity could take years before the [s] was correct in all contexts. The client would probably outgrow it before the clinician corrected it. This does not mean that shaping through successive approximation is not a valuable technique for the clinician. It only means that we need to make the process more efficient. Let us add modeling to our procedure.

Modeling

After the clinician has determined that the [s] is defective but before the client attempts to produce the sound, the clinician demonstrates the correct production for him. She produces the [s] sound in isolation and tells the client that this is his goal, to produce the sound as she made it for him. Now the client knows what the behavior change goal is and the clinician can now proceed with shaping through successive approximation. With each attempt that is closer to the correct production the clinician rewards him and then provides the model again. Our therapy is more efficient now but we can make it still more efficient by adding other techniques.

Guidance

After the clinician in our example has modeled the [s] sound for the client and has rewarded him for better productions, she reaches a point where the sound is not improving. The client is holding his lower lip too high and this is distorting the sound slightly. She might then say, "When you make the sound this time I am going to hold your lower lip down to where it should be when you make the [s] sound. Now listen to it again—[s]." When the client makes his next attempt the clinician holds the lower lip down slightly to improve the sound production. This is physical guidance. She is guiding him to improve the production of the sound. Our therapy is becoming more efficient but there are still other techniques we can add.

Information

The client is *blowing* too hard and it is distorting the sound production. The clinician adds behavior information about the sound production. She says to the client, "When you are making the sound don't blow the air out so hard. Blow the air out gently. Listen to me again—[s]." With information added to the model and guidance, the client again improves his sound production and is rewarded.

Reward/Token Economy

We began with shaping the behavior through rewards for behaviors that more closely approximated the correct behavior. We then added modeling, guidance, and information. Now, let us examine more carefully the reward itself and the procedure used to present the reward.

As the client is making attempts to produce the [s] sound, some of the attempts will more closely approximate the correct production. After each of these attempts, the clinician rewards him. She has decided that she will present a primary reward, a jelly bean, for each good production. If the client likes jelly beans, he will be motivated to produce the correct sound so that he can get them. This will increase the occurrence of the correct production. The clinician might be able to create even greater approach motivation if she rewarded him with two jelly beans.

If the clinician has decided to use a token economy she would give the client a token after each satisfactory production of the sound. She has some checkers in her desk which she uses as tokens. She first explains to the client that he would be able to buy some things from her "store" after therapy. She then shows him the things that she has for rewards. She might have, for example, some candy or small toys, each with a token price on it. After explaining this she initiates therapy, giving a token for good responses. After the therapy session is completed she opens the store and allows the client to purchase anything that he can afford. It is very important that the clinician have some items priced very low so that the client can always get some reward from the store. Again, two tokens might provide more approach motivation. The strength of the reward is indeed important.

Penalty

We have now dealt with rewarding good productions of the sound. How are we going to respond to those attempts the client makes that are not satisfactory? We have already discussed the disadvantages of trying to extinguish the behavior by not responding. Let us add another dimension to our therapy. Like trying to get a mule to move, we will not only dangle the reward of a carrot in front of him, we will also be behind him with a big stick in case he stops. Our clinical vehicle now has both front and rear wheel drive.

The clinician has been giving the client jelly beans for each good production of the [s] sound. She has the client save the jelly beans to eat after therapy so as to not interfere with the clinical process. They are in a small cup in front of the client. She now tells him that every time he makes the sound incorrectly, she is going to take back one jelly bean. If the jelly beans are really important to the client, he will make every effort possible to not lose any of them (just as you would do to avoid losing the $5 every time you were late to class or work). The clinician could increase the client's avoidance motivation by removing two jelly beans for each incorrect production. The strength of this penalty is directly related to how many jelly beans he receives for correct production. If he receives only one jelly bean, but loses two, there is an increase in avoidance motivation. Here we have another ratio that we can control. If he only loses one but gets two for correct production, we are focusing on approach motivation, but avoidance motivation is still a factor.

This same situation would exist if the clinician were using a token economy where she would remove a token for an incorrect production. She might increase the client's avoidance motivation to avoid the penalty if she removed two, or even three, tokens for an incorrect response. Our therapy now is doubly efficient. We are not only encouraging the correct responses through rewards, we are discouraging the incorrect responses through penalty. There are many variations the clinician can use in terms of the ratio or amount of reward and penalty in the token economy. If approach motivation is the key, the reward would consist of two tokens while the penalty would remain at one token. If the clinician wants to focus on avoidance motivation, the penalty could be two tokens and the reward one token. Approach motivation and avoidance motivation are different factors in therapy and the clinician may find herself using approach motivation during one phase of treatment and avoidance motivation in another.

When we are using rewards for the correct behavior and penalty for the incorrect behavior, our therapy is very efficient. Not only is the client trying to avoid the penalty by not producing the incorrect behavior, he is producing the correct behavior in order to get the reward. With this system, the correct behavior is being rewarded twice. The first reward is for the occurrence of the behavior while the second reward, a negative reward, is for the successful avoidance of the penalty. This is a very strong reward system. It is much stronger than only rewarding the correct productions and ignoring the incorrect productions. And when I say ignore the incorrect production, I mean just that. If a clinician is drilling a particular sound with a client and is presenting a token reward for each correct production and making no response to the incorrect productions, she is using a reward-oriented token economy. But, if she is giving tokens for correct productions and withholding the tokens for incorrect productions as well as telling the client that the production was wrong, she is using both rewards and penalties. Further, she is not just withholding a token, she is telling the client the production is wrong.

CLINICAL TRANSACTIONS: THE CIM

Initiating the First Transaction

Clinician to client. At this point in our therapy we have evaluated the client and determined what the problem is. We have also decided on the behavior change goal and have established rapport with our client. We are now ready to start the clinical process and teach the new behavior to the client. The first interaction between us and the client is the initial S—O—R. We are to present the first stimulus to the client. We have three choices of a stimulus as seen in Figure 5. We can provide any combination of modeling the behavior, guidance in the production of the behavior, or information about the behavior. Our choice of stimulus depends on what we hope to accomplish during our therapy session with the client and on any limitations our client might have such as lower cognitive functioning, a hearing problem, or visual problems.

If we are attempting to teach the client a behavior that can easily be seen and/or heard, we can use a model of the behavior. We may also want to include some information in this first contact with the client. Consider the following statement by a clinician, "We are going to learn to make the [s] sound today. It is a hissing sound, something like a snake makes. We hold our teeth close together, put the tongue up behind the teeth, and blow air out gently. Listen to me make the sound and then you try it—[s]." This clinician started the transaction by giving the client information about the sound and modeling it for him.

Another example might be the clinician working with an older client who stutters. The clinician has decided that she is going to work on the rate of speech. She could say, "Most people who stutter have a tendency to talk too fast. Research has shown that people who stutter do not have the same degree of fine motor skills as people who do not stutter. Speech is a fine motor skill and when the person who stutters talks too fast he is more likely to have the speech system break down. I am talking to you at the rate of speech I want you to imitate. Let me hear you count to 10 using this rate." Again, we have information and a model. This clinician might possibly decide to use a *delayed auditory feedback* (DAF) to get the client to slow down his rate. The DAF does not model slow speech for the stutterer but it does guide him to slower speech. To introduce this into therapy she could give the same information as before but then add, "This is a Delayed Auditory Feedback, a DAF. You will hear your own speech in the earphones I put on you but your speech will sound slower than you think it is. It will sound like an echo. You will have to talk slower when you are on the DAF. Now, let's put on the earphones and, when I signal, you count to 10."

When we make our choice of the stimulus to use in this initial contact, we must also consider the cognitive level of the client. If we present a model or information beyond the cognitive level of the client, it is inappropriate. The client will not comprehend what we are trying to teach. How do we determine the cognitive skills of the client? We should have some insight into his cognitive level from our initial evaluation. This first presentation is based on what we have already learned about the client's cognitive level but we may still present the stimuli at too complex a level. We will be adjusting our stimuli to the client's cognitive level during the first several transactions. This is part of the testing process that is included in each transaction.

Our testing of cognitive awareness and perception will be based on the resultant response of the client, the R in our diagram. If we present the [s] sound and the client produces a sound totally unrelated to the model, our test indicates that the model was probably inappropriate. Either the model was too complex or the client did not receive enough information from the model to reproduce it. It could also be that the client is responding too fast, not giving himself time to process the information he received from the model. We can slow down the response by telling him not to respond until we give him a signal of some sort.

If we then add information to the model and the same response occurs, the test again indicates that the stimulus we provided was not appropriate. We must continue to modify the stimulus until the client can comprehend it. The client's degree of comprehension is the core of the second half of the initial transaction.

Client to clinician. The response of the client is the stimulus for the clinician in the second half of our transaction. The model we are working on now is $S—O—R/\underline{S—O—R}$. This is the testing and decision making part of the transaction. The clinician perceived the client's response and evaluated it first in terms of correctness, completeness, and frequency of occurrence. If the response indicated that the client comprehended the initial stimulus and was able to produce an improved response, the clinician has established an appropriate level of stimulus for the client.

The clinician must then decide how she will respond to the client and what form of reward she will present. Of course, the reward should have been determined before the therapy began but some clinicians prefer to give spontaneous rewards. This preference is often the result of forgetting to plan therapy and the rewards usually take the form of verbal praise, such as "Very good, Johnny!" The major problem with this type of reward is how many times you can be told that you are doing a good job before it all becomes meaningless. Some clinicians use an abbreviated form of praise, simply saying "Good." This is even more meaningless. This form of "praise" even becomes meaningless to the clinician as she simply mouths the words. If the clinician observed the effect this reward has on the speech of the client she would realize that it is not an effective form of reward. It would be much more effective if the clinician combined her verbal praise with a token. The reward is very important for the approach motivation of the client. If the client is not interested in coming for therapy we are going to have clinical problems. One of the best rewards we can give a client is "fun" therapy. If a client is enjoying his therapy, does this mean that he is not learning anything? Therapy does not have to be tedious to be effective. If it is tedious it is because that is the way the clinician views therapy.

If the client's response was not satisfactory, the clinician must reevaluate her stimuli and also respond in some way. Because this is the first transaction, the penalty, if given, should be carefully adjusted in terms of its strength. In other words, be gentle. The clinician might possibly respond by saying, "You made a good try." This rewards the effort the client made but also tells him that the response was not satisfactory. It is too early in therapy to focus on the avoidance motivation of the client. In the early part of therapy our approach should be as positive as possible. Nevertheless, we will encounter clients where we have to focus on the client's avoidance motivation early in therapy. This is especially true for those clients for whom we are unable to find an appropriate reward. These clients are few and far between, but they do exist.

Since we are still in the first clinical transaction, the effect of the reward or the penalty has not had an opportunity to influence either the frequency of occurrence of the speech behavior or the attending behaviors of the client. We need to sit down and think through our clinical approach very carefully if we have lost the client this early in therapy! We will begin monitoring the influences of the reward and penalty after therapy has progressed a bit further.

Before concluding the first transaction the clinician must decide what her next stimulus will be to initiate the second transaction. If the initial stimulus did not achieve the desired results and the client's response was not satisfactory, the next stimulus must be modified. The model must be made slower and clearer. More information could be provided to clarify the behavior for the client. The clinician might even decide to add guidance to the stimulus. It is possible to combine all three stimuli in introducing the next transaction. It would be feasible for the clinician to combine them in this way: "When you just made the [s] sound your lower lip was too high and the sound could not get out. When you make it this time, I am going to hold your lower lip down so the sound can get out. Now, listen and watch me make the sound and then you try it again—[s]." She then holds the lower lip down while the client makes the next attempt. She has used modeling, guidance, and information. If she must modify this stimulus even more in the future she can expand the amount of information by explaining the sound production more carefully, exaggerate the production of the model of the sound, and exert even more guidance on the lower lip.

When the client's response is satisfactory at this step of shaping, the clinician then moves ahead in therapy. She provides a stimulus that moves the behavioral production to the next step in successive approximation.

Initiating the Second Transaction

As you can see in the CIM, the clinician has determined the stimulus and the direction of the next transaction before the first transaction is completed. She then terminates the first transaction with her response and starts the next one with her stimulus. For example, the clinician might say, "That was a pretty good sound, David, but I think you can do it better" (response–penalty). "Now, watch me again. I will do it slower this time so you can see exactly how I do it. Watch how I hold my teeth together–[ssss]" (stimulus–information and model). The second transaction is now underway with the client perceiving the stimulus, thinking about it, and then responding. If the client's response is too fast, it can be slowed down by introducing a signal for the client to respond. The efficiency of therapy is not dependent on the speed of the client's response. The clinician again evaluates the response, decides how she will respond, and determines her stimulus to initiate the next transaction. The transactions now continue with the clinician and the client playing their respective roles.

As the transactions continue, the clinician becomes more involved in monitoring the second transactional mode, the effects of the reward and penalty on the frequency of occurrence of speech behaviors, and on the approach motivation and/or avoidance motivation of the client. These factors become more influential as the client has extended experience with the reward and the penalty. He must develop approach motivation to get the reward and avoidance motivation to avoid the penalty. This is another part of the cognitive function of the client in therapy.

Ongoing Transactions

Therapy is now underway. Each transaction builds on the preceding one. The clinician uses shaping to bring the behavior, through steps of successive approximation, closer and closer to the behavior change goal. She continues to model, give information, and give guidance as the behavior changes. The better productions of the behavior are rewarded while the poorer productions are penalized. She is using a constant reward schedule because it results in quicker learning. As the behavior begins to stabilize she fades the model, information, and guidance until the behavior occurs without assistance. She continues to monitor the second transactional mode, keeping track of the client's attentiveness and frequency of occurrence of the speech behaviors. She may have to adjust her reward and/or penalty, but this can be done quickly so that therapy can proceed. We complete this step in the clinical process when the behavior occurs spontaneously or through a gestural prompt. We are still rewarding each occurrence but there is no penalty since the behavior is stable and production errors no longer occur.

Keep in mind that we have two basic modes of clinical transactions, one being focused on *speech* behavior and the other on *attending* behavior. If the client is attending to therapy, and the speech behavior is responding appropriately to either reward or penalty, the attending behavior is only monitored as therapy progresses. However, if a problem arises in terms of the client's attending to therapy, the transactions shift to the secondary mode where the focus is on the attending behavior. We can improve the client's attending to therapy either through his approach motivation or his avoidance motivation.

STIMULUS MANIPULATION

Role Shift

In this early stage of treatment we are not going to be concerned with all three categories of stimuli (people, talking situations, and objects). We are going to concentrate on shifting stimulus roles of the various people in our client's nonclinical environments. Obviously there are going to be many instances in therapy where we will not have an opportunity to work either directly or indirectly with significant others in our client's lives. This lack is going to have an adverse effect on our therapy in that the client does not have a "support system" as he goes through therapy. But, this is a fact of life.

If we were able to work with the significant others, it might be worthwhile to consider their stimulus roles before we come in contact with the client. Regardless of the type of communication disorder, the significant others were either rewarding the communication disorder or penalizing it. They either had a positive or negative reaction to the disorder. In either event, it would be wise to minimize this influence before treatment begins. It would be difficult to

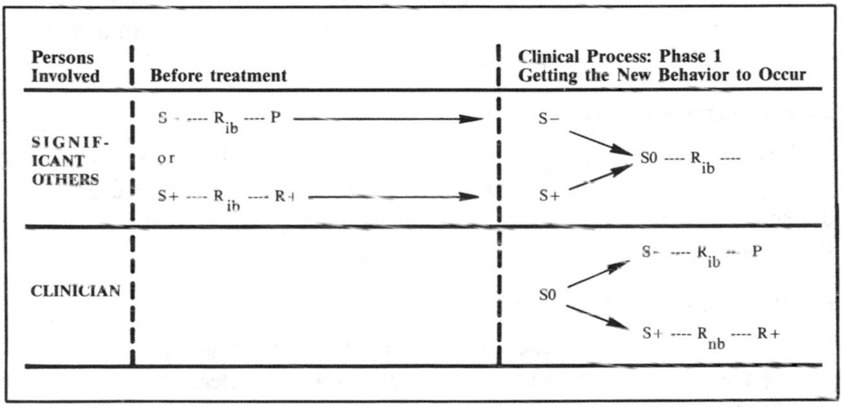

FIGURE 8
Stimulus Role Shift Model—Clinical Process: Phase 1. Before treatment the significant others either directly or indirectly reward or penalize the incorrect behavior. Their stimulus roles are then either an S+ (reward) or an S– (penalty). The clinician is not yet involved with the client or the significant others. As treatment starts, Phase 1, the influence of the significant others is neutralized by shifting their stimulus roles from an S+ or an S– to an S0, neither rewarding nor penalizing the incorrect behavior. The clinician shifts her stimulus role from a neutral stimulus, S0, to an S+, rewarding the new behavior, and an S–, penalizing the incorrect behavior.

penalize an incorrect behavior in the clinical environment while it was being rewarded in the home. As is shown in Figure 8, the significant other's role is shifted to that of an S0. There is no way we can completely eliminate all positive or negative reactions made by the significant others; but we can reduce them and their effect through counseling, and telling them how to respond in a more neutral manner.

At the same time, as therapy beings, the clinician shifts from her S0 role before therapy to that of an S+ for the new behavior and an S- for the old behavior. Her role shift is accomplished through her association with the rewards and penalties.

Gradual Introduction of Stimuli

The gradual introduction of stimuli has little value at this stage of therapy. It would only apply to such things as a gradual increase in the amount of information we might use as part of the stimulus, or a gradual increase in the amount of physical guidance we provide a client. This form of manipulation will be important in later stages of therapy.

Gradual Withdrawal of Stimuli

Gradual withdrawal of stimuli is an important function in that we must gradually withdraw or "fade" the stimuli used to create the new behavior. As the behavior becomes more stable we can fade the model, the information, and the guidance. We can fade all at the same time or we can fade one at a time. Fading may involve decreasing the frequency of occurrence of guidance, the intensity or strength of a model, the duration or completeness of information, or any combination with any stimuli.

Increase the Number of Stimuli

This stimulus manipulation method is not extremely important in this therapy phase. The only way we use it is when we add guidance and then information to the model. We increase the number of stimuli that make up the stimulus we use to initiate each clinical transaction.

Decreasing the Number of Stimuli

At this early stage of therapy we are limited to decreasing the number of S+ and S- that are associated with the communication disorder. This is limited to shifting the roles of the significant others in the client's most immediate environment.

CLINICAL EXAMPLES

Now that we have covered all of the pertinent information regarding the CIM model, let us take time to consider several clinical examples. We will take several clients and adjust the CIM model to the particular client by manipulating the antecedent events. We will then consider other clients where we will have to manipulate contingent events to the unique needs of the client. If you see some factors that should have been considered, but which I overlooked, remember that "To err is human, to forgive, divine."

Manipulating the Antecedent Events

Example 1. Our client is an 8-year-old female with a high-frequency hearing loss and a resultant distortion of the sibilants. It is our decision to begin work on the [s] sound. We normally model the sound for the client and see if the client can imitate the sound. However, we recognize that the high-frequency hearing loss may prevent the client from perceiving the model correctly. This does not mean that we cannot use the auditory channel. We can still use it for behavioral information. We can use the model of the sound but it will be aimed primarily at the visual channel so that the client can see the articulatory position to assume for the correct production. We then supplement the model with behavioral information concerning the placement of the articulators. Information concerning the "quality" of the sound is not appropriate here because of the hearing problem. The client really does not know how a snake sounds. If this stimuli is not sufficient to produce a better [s] sound we can also introduce physical guidance for the articulatory position. In this instance we might use a tongue blade to provide physical guidance of the lips and positioning of the teeth. Fingers are frowned on in most clinical settings. Bites can be painful. With each presentation of the stimuli we shape the production of the [s] sound. Although the client may not be able to hear the subtle changes we make in the [s] production, she will be able to discern the physical changes in the positioning of the articulators. In this particular instance we modify our behavior change goal from a "perfect" [s] production to an "acceptable" one because there is an organic factor involved in the error. The physical monitoring of the production by the client is not as accurate and reliable as auditory monitoring would be. We have now adjusted our stimuli to the limitations of the client, utilizing as much of the auditory channel as is practical and supplementing it with the visual and body sense channels.

Example 2. This client is a 7-year-old male who omits the [ɝ] sound. One of the problems in teaching this sound is that the unique tongue position for the sound is not visible. If we open our mouth wide during the production of the sound so that the client can see it, the tongue position and the sound itself are distorted. Thus, the model is somewhat limited in terms of visual information concerning the placement of the tongue. In order to expand the stimuli we would add behavioral information, telling the client where to put his tongue and how to hold it. Again, we might provide physical guidance with a tongue blade to help the client get the tongue where it should be. Another type of guidance might be verbal guidance where we tell the client to make the sound of a fire engine. The client might be able to produce the [ɝ] sound in this context but not when asked to produce the sound as a phoneme. If the fire engine fails, try a police car.

Example 3. We are faced with an adult male client with expressive aphasia and severe apraxia. He cannot voluntarily control any of his articulators. He cannot even open his mouth upon command. For all intents and purposes the client is nonverbal, although he makes grunting sounds which appear to have no significance. Our evaluation indicates that he comprehends at a relatively normal level. The first task we set for ourselves is to increase voluntary control over the articulators and we are going to start on opening the mouth. We model the behavior and the client struggles but cannot perform the behavior. We then verbally request the client to open his mouth as we model the behavior. Again, the client attempts to follow the instructions but is unable to do so. Because this is an apraxia, we know that behaviors can occur on a reflex level even though they cannot be performed voluntarily. What can we use to elicit a reflexive opening of the mouth? With some clinicians I have observed, their being prepared for a therapy session would trigger this response; but the most obvious stimulus which would trigger this mouth opening would seem to be a spoon. Turning to environmental guidance, we take the spoon and place it at the client's mouth. The client's mouth opens reflexively to receive food. We now have the behavior occurring but we need to change the stimulus which cues the behavior from the spoon to the verbal request. We then pair the verbal request with the presentation of the spoon saying, "Open your mouth" as the spoon is moved toward the mouth. We now begin to gradually withdraw the presentation of the spoon (fading this stimulus) as we continue to make the verbal request. After the association is made between the verbal request and the mouth opening, the response will occur without the spoon being present. In this instance we had to bypass the purely cognitive approach and start from a reflex level in order to get the behavior to occur.

Example 4. Let us consider another adult aphasic client. There is no apraxia with this female client but there is a severe expressive aphasia. She has some expressive language but has difficulty naming objects. This is a transient problem since many times she can recall the names of objects. This tells us that simply modeling the name of an object is useless since she already knows the name and how to say it. She just cannot recall the name at various times. We need to develop another cue that will assist the client in remembering the name when her normal recall procedures fail her. We decide that the word we want to work on is "cup." We bring a cup into therapy with us and, as we model the word for her to repeat, we have her look at the cup and pick it up as if to drink some coffee. We are now building associations between the word and the visual and motor cues. We can then gradually withdraw the model and introduce verbal guidance in the form of a question such as, "What do you drink coffee from?" We must be careful how we phrase the question. If we asked, "How do you drink your coffee?" the client might respond, "With cream and sugar." If the natural recall process fails here as she attempts to answer the question, she is able to look at the cup for additional cuing information. If this fails to cue the word, she can then pick up the cup as if to drink some coffee. She is adding still another cuing system to aid her recall of the word. We have now taught her to add visual and body sense cues to supplement the natural word recall process.

Example 5. This client is an 18-year-old female stutterer. Our clinical goal is to reduce her speaking rate in order to achieve fluency. We first of all try modeling the rate of speech that we want along with some behavioral information about how to speak slower. We find that even with the model, information, and verbal guidance in the form of cues or hints about the speech rate, the client is unable to slow her speech rate. We then put the client on a Delayed Auditory Feedback (DAF) where she hears her speech through earphones only after a .25-second delay. After some initial faltering, she begins to speak at a very slow rate. This is environmental guidance. We have manipulated her auditory environment in such a way that slow speech rate is elicited. The DAF forces the slower rate of speech. We must now slowly remove the DAF as the behavior is maintained. We can do this by gradually reducing the amount of delay in the speech playback. This is a unique form of environmental guidance in that it is a clinical instrument that "elicits" or forces a response of slow speech. In this instance, we are changing the input signal in such a way that the speech rate is reduced. It is the output of the DAF, the delayed feedback, that provides the changed speech signal which produces the change in rate. In this way the DAF is a stimulus, an environmental guidance stimulus.

Manipulating the Contingent Events

Example 1. Our client in this example is a 5-year-old male with a slight articulation disorder. When the client first came in for therapy he paid close attention to the therapy and seemed to enjoy his time with us. He made good progress on his speech and he was rewarded with colored stars which were stuck on his work papers. However, as the novelty of the clinical experience wore off, the child gradually began to lose interest in therapy. He would daydream during therapy and clinical progress was digressing. We were aware of both types of clinical transactions, speech behavior and attending behavior, and, although we had been focusing on the speech behavior transactions, we were monitoring the attending behaviors. As the client's attending behaviors began to fade, we recognized that the efficiency of our therapy was also fading. We could not teach him if he was not paying attention. In order to correct this situation we shifted our clinical focus to the attending behavior transactions. The first thing we have to recognize is that our reward is no longer actually rewarding to the client. He has received so many stars that they no longer have value to him. So we either have to change our reward in order to achieve approach motivation or introduce a penalty to achieve avoidance motivation. Both approach motivation and avoidance motivation will get the attending behavior for us. How do we decide which will be more effective? Let us first consider that things went very well in therapy until the reward lost its value. The easiest thing to do would be to find another form of reward. We are working with eight other children in this agency and several of them have also tired of their rewards. So, we decide to use a token economy on all of our clients. We gather a number of what we hope are interesting items which could serve as rewards. We have trinkets, gum, candy, and various small toys. We keep these "goodies" in a container. This, then, constitutes our "store." The first day we change over to the token economy we make sure that each client gets some tokens and then we open up our store for them. When they make their first purchase, the association is made between the tokens and the backup rewards. Now they are hooked. There are so many things to choose from! They would like several things but they can only afford one item each time the store is open. Then there is "inflation." Clinicians soon learn to set the prices high enough so that they are not spending half their salary on rewards. With this reward system, we have greatly reduced the chances of our client losing interest in his rewards. There is a wide variety of rewards available and he gets his choice of the one that is most important to him.

We now shift our clinical focus to attending behaviors and, when the client is attending, we give him a token. The token might be given to him for a correct response to a model but the correct response indicates that he was attending. With his increased interest in achieving the reward we now have approach motivation to perform the behaviors that will be rewarded. Once we have regained the client's attending behavior and approach motivation, we can shift back to the speech behavior transactions, but we will continue to monitor the client's attending behavior.

Example 2. We are now faced with a 16-year-old female client who has severe language delay, possibly a working vocabulary of 35 words, 20 of which cannot be printed in this book. Her comprehension is good even though the records indicate rather extensive brain injury at birth. The client is emotionally impaired and demonstrates aggressive behavior toward teachers and therapists. On the first day of therapy we took her into the clinic room and started our first clinical transaction. Her response was to spit on us. Each time we would present her with a stimulus, her response was to spit. Should we try to extinguish the behavior by ignoring it? How do you ignore someone who is spitting on you? Obviously we cannot start therapy until this behavior is dealt with. We must deal directly with this behavior by finding a contingent event that influences the frequency of occurrence of the spitting. Our client finds the behavior itself rewarding so we must find a penalty that is stronger than the reward she is experiencing. The first thing we try is spitting back at her (crude, perhaps, but practical). She enjoys this (it is a reward), and her spitting increases in frequency. We then decide that when she spits we will hold her hands firmly in her lap for one minute. When we do this, the client becomes quite agitated. We carefully explain that if she spits on us we will hold her hands in her lap for a period of time. We now find that the occurrence of spitting behavior is lessening. The client is developing avoidance motivation toward the unpleasant experience of having her hands held in her lap. Our clinical role is changing with the client. She has associated us with the penalty for spitting. We have become an S– for the spitting behavior. When she sees us she is cued that if the spitting occurs she will be penalized. So, in our presence, there is no longer any spitting behavior. However, the spitting behavior will continue to occur at the same level in other environments where there is no S– to cue the penalty. We can now move on to basic treatment procedures with this client.

Example 3. We are now going to deal with a 35-year-old male stutterer. Our clinical goal is to establish a slower rate of speech but we do not have to use a DAF. He is able to follow the model of rate we are providing. We are going to start shaping his speech rate by rewarding his speech when it approximates the speech rate we want. In our conversations with the client we are careful to model the desired rate of speech. When he answers us we will determine if his speech rate is closer to our model and, if so, he is rewarded. However, there are many instances where his speech rate is much too fast. In order to make our therapy more efficient, we decide that we are not going to ignore these fast speech episodes, we are going to penalize them. Our main problem now is to create appropriate rewards and penalties for an adult. If the way to a man's heart is through his stomach, the way to his approach motivation and avoidance motivation is through his wallet. We have the client bring in $2 in dimes, and we set up the contingencies. Each time he produces a slower rate of speech that approximates our model, he get $.20 back. Every time he speaks too fast, he loses $.10. The client now has a great deal of approach motivation to get back his $2 by performing at the correct rate. He also has the avoidance motivation to avoid losing his money by speaking too fast. What does he substitute for his fast talking? Slow talking. The slow talking then is directly rewarded by his receiving $.20 and negatively rewarded by his not losing $.10. This particular arrangement is biased toward the reward side of the economy. Then, later in therapy, our client becomes a bit lazy. He can receive four rewards and this will cancel out eight penalties (a little exercise in higher math). We want to stress the elimination of the fast rate of speech so we change the economy so that each episode of slow talking is rewarded by $.10 but each instance of fast talking is penalized by the loss of $.30. We have now reversed the focal point of the economy. We are now concentrating on the penalty, providing the client with much avoidance motivation to avoid losing his money. The approach motivation is still operating ($.10 worth) but the prime mover is the avoidance motivation to avoid losing $.30 each time the rate is too fast.

As this is all transpiring, we are assuming new roles in the clinic room. When we are rewarding proper rate, we assume the role of S+, cuing this behavior to occur. As we penalize the fast rate we become an S–, cuing the faster speech not to occur. In order to maintain these roles we must continue to reward and penalize. This creates no problem since we are in the phase of therapy where we are using constant reward when the correct behavior occurs and constant penalty when the fast rate occurs.

PLANNING AND PROBLEM SOLVING

The following clinical situations are for you to ponder. Each will pose a problem in either planning an appropriate stimulus, selecting an appropriate reward/penalty system, or solving a problem encountered in an ongoing clinical interaction. Review each situation carefully and then write down your analysis of the situation and what you would do. After you have finished all of the clinical situations, turn to Appendix C where each situation is discussed. These discussions are not meant to be "the answers" but rather a discussion of important points to consider and possible solutions. There are no single solutions to these situations. But, as someone once said, "Two heads are better than one."

Situation A

The evaluation of this 17-year-old male indicates that he is rather severely retarded in terms of language skills. Even the limited vocabulary is difficult to understand because of poor motor control over the articulatory system. The history indicates brain injury at birth and general mental retardation. An audiological report states that the client could not be adequately tested but there appears to be a rather significant hearing loss in both ears. The client is in a foster care facility where he must be able to let his needs and wants be known. The problem is that he has neither the vocabulary nor the articulatory skills to communicate his needs. Your task is to create a clinical program such that you can teach this client a basic needs vocabulary that other people can understand. You should concentrate your planning on an appropriate stimulus system for this client.

Situation B

Your client is a 45-year-old male who has recently had a laryngectomy. He is discouraged about ever learning to talk again. You have this client in individual therapy three days a week. Your task is to teach him to use esophageal speech. Your primary focus should be on the types of stimuli you are going to use with this client. Also discuss the ways you might use contingent events with this client.

Situation C

This client is a 7-year-old female with an articulation disorder. There is nothing significant about the girl except that she comes from a wealthy family who have doted on her every whim. In nontechnical language she is spoiled rotten. If there is something she does not have it is only because she does not want it. You must plan your contingencies around this.

Situation D

This 9-year-old boy has a rather severe voice disorder. He has had an examination by a physician who reported that he has vocal nodes. Your evaluation indicated that a good share of the vocal abuse was due to his use of sudden vocal onset (hard vocal attack or onset) as part of his speech. How would you teach this new vocal behavior to the client? How would you introduce other factors involved in vocal abuse?

Chapter 5

Synopsis

We have now progressed to the point where the new behavior is occurring consistently in the clinical environment although it is still dependent on prompts or cues and the reward. We now need to stabilize it and make it independent of prompts, cues, and rewards. The behavior must be habituated in the clinical environment before we can generalize it to other environments. We must gradually wean the behavior from the prompts, cues, and rewards and then test it to see if it is stable and habituated. This chapter will discuss how this is achieved in this phase of therapy.

Chapter 5

Habituating the
New Behavior

ANTECEDENT AND CONTINGENT
EVENTS IN THE CIM

At this phase of the clinical process the new behavior is stable in the clinic room but it is still somewhat dependent on prompts or cues and the reward. We have continued with a constant reward program up to this point in therapy. If you get the feeling that this step overlaps with the last step, you are right. It is very hard to differentiate between the last stages of getting the behavior to occur and the first stages of habituating the behavior. There is no clear line of demarcation, no clear-cut border. But, we will be using different strategies in this step so we will discuss it as a separate phase of therapy. Our task here is to make the behavior independent of the prompts, cues, and rewards.

The focus in this phase of therapy is on the contingent events. The reward schedule we have used up to this point was designed for quick learning. But, with a constant schedule of reward, when the reward is removed the behavior quickly extinguishes. In this phase of the clinical process we must change the schedule to intermittent rewards. With this schedule, behaviors become very stable and quite independent of the reward. It is almost impossible to extinguish a behavior that has been learned on an intermittent reward schedule. When we use this reward schedule our client never knows when he is going to receive a reward. He may perform the behavior three times with no reward and then on the fourth time he gets the reward. He continues to perform the behavior, waiting for the reward. This practice of the behavior without the reward is the important part of habituation. Many people in our society have been "trained" to perform a specific behavior with this type of reward schedule. It is known as gambling and the most obvious example is the slot machine. You put in five coins with no reward and then with the sixth coin you receive four coins back. Unless your math is extremely poor, you recognize that you are still two coins short. But, do you stop? No, you are encouraged to play more coins in the hope that you will receive another reward, maybe even the Jackpot. So, you put back the four coins you received plus five more before you are rewarded again. This time you are paid off with 15 coins and you are 6 coins ahead. This is obviously the time to stop playing. However, there is that human element called greed and this keeps most people playing. Being human, you also keep playing. You do not stop and think about your chances of winning, you only know that there is a chance that you will "win big." Of course, in this example we have two factors operating, intermittent reward and greed. If you have ever been to a gambling casino you have probably noticed people who sit between two slot machines and play them for hours on end, perhaps even days on end. They are "hooked." Intermittent reward is a powerful learning tool.

Fading Antecedent Events

If you will recall, we had a series of antecedent events which we used to get the new behavior to occur. We faded or withdrew most of these events toward the end of the previous phase of therapy. The model was no longer needed. But we did continue to use environmental, verbal, and gestural guidance to prompt the new behavior to occur. We did things like show the client pictures that would prompt the behavior, verbally request the behavior, or gesture in such a way that the client would perform the behavior. The behavior did not yet occur spontaneously.

Now we want to withdraw these cues so that the behavior occurs spontaneously. For example, instead of using pictures that are aimed directly at prompting the behavior such as a picture of a snake for the [s] sound or a cup to prompt the word, we would use more subtle cues. We might use a general picture with many objects and see if the [s] sound occurs or we could use a saucer and see if the word "cup" is produced. This same process would be applied to verbal and gestural cues. They are modified to more subtle forms. Once the behavior is occurring with these subtle prompts, we can remove the prompts and the behavior will occur spontaneously. The withdrawal process must be gradual, allowing the client to adjust to more subtle cues.

Fading the Contingent Events

Let us first of all consider the role of penalty in the habituation of the new behavior. Penalty plays a minor role if it plays any role at all. We have established the behavior in the previous step of therapy and the error is no longer occurring. Therefore, we no longer need to penalize incorrect productions. However, in some clinical instances, we might have to incorporate penalty to a minor degree. If we are working with a client who has an articulation problem and we are incorporating the new sound into words, we may have to back up a bit in the clinical process to get the new sound to occur in specific words as we are habituating. In this instance we would use penalty. So, let us not totally abandon the concept of penalty in this step of therapy. As the error occurs less often, the penalty will be faded.

The gradual withdrawal of the reward is extremely important. In the previous phase of therapy we were rewarding each and every performance of the behavior. Now, if we suddenly take away the reward, the behavior will extinguish. It will gradually disappear. We must change the schedule of presentation of the reward. When we shift to an intermittent reward schedule we have several choices on how to do this. We can base our presentation of the reward on either the number of times the behavior is performed before it is rewarded (ratio system) or we can use time as a factor (interval system). If we are using the number of times the behavior is performed we will be using the ratio system. If we decide on a fixed ratio, we decide that the client will receive a reward after an exact number of performances. If we have a ratio of 3:1, this means that he receives the reward on the fourth performance. There is also the variable ratio. This means that we do not stick to a constant number of performances before giving the reward. The client might perform the behavior two times and receive a reward and then perform it five times before the next reward. The system is constantly varying according to the clinician.

With time being the base for the reward schedule we again have two choices, the fixed interval and the variable interval. The fixed interval means that we reward the client after a standard period of time while the variable interval calls for rewards being presented according to variable intervals of time.

In my clinical experience I have found that the time base is not practical for most speech behaviors. What do you do if, within the time interval you have selected, the client does not perform the behavior? This type of schedule does not appear to fit the general needs of the speech clinician. However, if you are attempting to increase the duration of a behavior such as paying attention or sitting in a chair, the time base is ideal. The fixed and variable interval systems of reward presentation have a unique application for the speech clinician. We will be using the fixed and variable ratio schedules in most of our therapy. I have used both and found that they both work very well in therapy. My main problem with the fixed ratio was that I had to keep counting the number of times the client performed the behavior so that I could reward him. Because counting distracts my attention from therapy, I shifted to the variable ratio and found that I was very comfortable with it.

With either of the ratio schedules, however, it is important that the reward occur less and less often as habituation occurs. With the fixed ratio schedule, the ratio would have to increase over time. The clinician might start with a 3:1 ratio but then have to shift to 4:1, then 5:1, and so on. With the variable ratio schedule the clinician would have to make sure that the number of performances increases before the reward is given. Eventually, if the client receives a reward after 20 performances, the behavior is not dependent on the reward and the reward can be completely removed.

TESTING HABITUATION

If the reward is removed and the behavior continues to occur, it is habituated. You might view this as an indication that the behavior itself has become rewarding. In any event, after the reward that we provide the client has been removed and the behavior continues to occur, the behavior has been habituated and will occur spontaneously with no prompts and no reward from the clinician. But what are we going to do if, when we remove the reward, the behavior begins to falter? We must go back to our reward schedule at a level where the behavior is occurring again. Once we have the behavior stable at this level, we reinstate the withdrawal program. What did all of this tell us? It told us that we moved too quickly in the removal of the reward. If "patience is a virtue," then all speech clinicians must be virtuous.

STIMULUS MANIPULATION

Role Shift

As we move into the second phase of the clinical process we are still going to concentrate on the people in the client's environments. We also begin to consider the other types of stimuli, talking situations and objects. Let us consider each of these in order.

Significant others and the clinician. It is now time to shift the significant other's role from that of an S0 established while the new behavior was being created to that of an S+ for the new behavior and an S– for the old behavior. This is done so that the generalization process can begin. This is accomplished by having the significant others begin to reward the new behavior when it occurs in the external environment and to penalize the old behavior when it occurs (see Figure 9). This process of shifting roles should not be done immediately but should occur while the client is still in this phase of the clinical process. The clinician must carefully identify for the significant others what the new behavior is, determine what the reward will be, and how often the reward is presented. If a token system is employed, the type of token reward and the backup rewards must be determined. It is also important that the significant others start with a constant reward schedule so that the new behavior is encouraged to occur in the external environment.

As the roles of the significant others are shifting, the clinician is also shifting her roles. In the previous step she had been an S+ for the new behavior and an S– for the old behavior. The old behavior was occurring less and less so the need for penalty diminished. As this occurred, the clinician's role of S– faded but the role of S+ was even stronger since she was rewarding all occurrences and, by the end of this step, all occurrences were correct. She now begins to withdraw the reward by changing the schedule of reward from a constant schedule to an intermittent schedule. When the new behavior occurs and the clinician does not reward it, she begins to assume the role of S0. The role of S0 becomes more

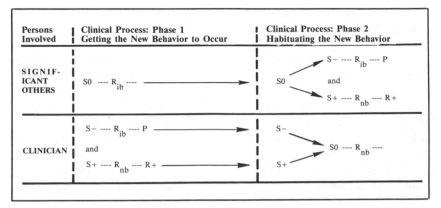

FIGURE 9
Stimulus Role Shift Model—Clinical Process: Phase 2. As treatment progresses from Phase 1 to Phase 2, the significant others' stimulus roles are shifted from that of an S0 to an S+, rewarding the new behavior, and an S−, penalizing the incorrect behavior in order to encourage the new behavior to begin to occur in the external environment. To test the habituation of the new behavior in the clinical environment, the clinician shifts her stimulus roles from S+ and S− to that of an S0. In doing this she removes the contingent rewards to test the stability of the new behavior.

and more pronounced as the ratio of reward changes. When the ratio is 1:1 she is an S0 half of the time but when the ratio is 5:1 the role of S0 occurs 80% of the time. In this way the clinician slowly assumes the role of S0, testing the habituation of the new behavior in the clinical environment.

Other stimuli. In many instances it will be very important for us to begin shifting the roles of other stimuli, talking situations, and objects while the therapy is still centered in the clinical environment. This does not apply to all clients, but only those where the S− are so strong that the client will need direct assistance in dealing with them. The factor that determines whether or not we will start role shifting in this phase of therapy seems to be the emotional involvement of the client with both his disorder and the stimuli. We will want to begin the role shift in the clinical environment since we will have maximum control over the stimuli. Once the client is working alone in the external environment, our control over the stimuli is greatly reduced and the client may not be able to perform the new speech behavior when confronted with the stimuli. Within the clinical environment, we can manipulate the stimuli in ways to encourage the new speech behavior to occur. We might view this early role shifting as a "halfway house" for the client. He is being provided with a means to deal with the S− situations in a controlled environment. This experience will increase the probability that he will be able to deal with the S− situations in the external environment.

Talking situations. It might be important to start working on role shifts for talking situations while still in this step in the clinical process. This would be particularly true for those clients who stutter. If a certain situation is an S– for the client it could be dealt with initially in the clinical environment where the clinician has control over the "strength" of the situation. She could begin to change the role of this situation through gradual introduction of the stimulus. This would include such talking situations as speaking before groups or talking to clerks in stores. The gradual introduction of the stimuli could be accomplished through techniques such as "role playing," "sociodramas," or whatever name is used to describe the process of creating situations in the clinic room that give the client an opportunity to practice his new speech behaviors in a controlled environment. Role shifting of talking situations in this step in therapy is usually reserved for special clients with special needs. It is not the rule, it is the exception.

Objects. As with talking situations, objects may need to be dealt with within the clinical environment. Objects that have the role of S– might include the telephone, dictating machines, tape recorders, public address systems, and other such communication devices. Object fear is usually associated with clients who stutter. It is often advisable to deal initially with these objects in the controlled clinical environment as a form of prelude to generalizing the new behavior, the next step in our therapy. Gradual presentation of the stimulus object is used to begin to change the role of the object. With the telephone, the clinician might start with the easiest telephone situation and then gradually increase the difficulty. The first task the client might have would be to look at a "dead" telephone (a disconnected telephone) while remaining calm. When the client can do this, he would touch the telephone, maintaining his composure. The next step would be to put the receiver to his ear. Following steps would include dialing the telephone and asking for a specific person. This same process is used with other objects. It is "role playing" with feared objects.

Gradual Introduction of Stimuli

It is evident from role shifting that this form of stimulus manipulation is used selectively in this step of therapy. Its use is limited to those S– stimuli that need to be dealt with in the clinical environment. We will not use this form of manipulation of talking situations and objects with all types of clients.

As we are changing the roles of the significant others to S+ and S– as discussed above, we gradually introduce these new stimuli to the client. This is a gradual process as the significant others become associated with rewards and penalties for specific behaviors. Also, as the clinician shifts her role from a strong S+ to an S0, this new role is gradually introduced.

Gradual Withdrawal of Stimuli

There is only limited use of this form of manipulation in this step in therapy. The clinician gradually withdraws rewards as the schedule of rewards changes. This results in the gradual withdrawal of the S+ role of the clinician. We also gradually withdraw the S0 role of the significant others as they assume their new roles of S+ and S−.

Increasing the Number of Stimuli

The stimuli we are dealing with here are the significant others. As we shift their roles we are increasing the number of S+ for the new speech behavior and increasing the number of S− for the old behavior. Prior to this, the only S+ and S− the client associated with his speech was the clinician. It is possible that the talking situations and objects that the clinician worked on in the clinical environment have also shifted their roles, and in this event we would also be increasing the number of S+ to cue the new behavior. However, this role shift might still be limited to the clinic room since the client has not dealt with the stimuli in the external environment.

Decreasing the Number of Stimuli

You have probably recognized by now that we are dealing with two types of S−. We are using one form of S− to discourage the occurrence of the old behavior and we are increasing the number of these stimuli. But we also have S− roles associated with specific talking situations and objects. These S− are indirectly associated with the incorrect speech behavior. They cue a negative emotional response in the client which interferes with the performance of the new speech behavior. We need to decrease the number of these S− in order for the client to be able to perform the new speech behavior in their presence. We accomplish this shift of the role of the stimuli through gradual introduction of the stimuli in the clinical environment.

CLINICAL EXAMPLES

Fading the Antecedent Events

Example 1. Our client in this example is a 10-year-old male who is nonverbal. We have taught him to say the word "water" in the previous step in therapy. The antecedent events we used were the model of the word and environmental guidance in the form of pictures of a lake and a glass of water. We used a token economy as a reward system. We started out by giving him a drink of water after each production of the word but we ran into two problems. First of all he became satiated with water and second our therapy was constantly interrupted with his having to go to the bathroom. So we shifted to tokens which he could use to purchase a drink of water when he wanted it. In the habituation step of therapy we would begin to fade the visual cues by using pictures that would include some aspect of water but not as a main theme. We might use a picture of a kitchen sink and a picture of a boat. We then gradually fade this type of cue, changing perhaps to taking the client to a sink and seeing if this environmental cue elicits the response.

Example 2. This client is a 15-year-old stutterer. We have established a slower rate of speech using the DAF. He is now speaking at the new rate while on the DAF, even though there is no delay in the speech signal he hears since we have faded the delay from .25 seconds to .0-second delay. In other words, he is hearing himself normally through the DAF. We then begin to turn down the volume of the DAF so that eventually he can hear nothing through the earphones. The next step is to remove the earphones as he continues to talk at the new rate. We then move the DAF unit to another part of the clinic room. The final step is to remove the DAF from the clinical room.

Fading the Contingent Events

In that we are dealing with a single event in this section, we are limited to the number of clinical examples we can discuss since they would all be the same. We are only concerned with the frequency of presentation of the reward, regardless of whether we are using ratios or intervals. If we withdraw the reward too fast, the behavior may begin to extinguish. We must then go back and provide rewards more often. Let us consider a single example and see if you can generalize it to all types of clients. In this example we are dealing with a 7-year-old female client who has been taught the [k] sound in words. The reward has been green stars which are stuck in her speech book behind the words she has been working on. We now change to red stars so we can tell which stars have been given for each step in therapy. We use a variable ratio for the reward, being careful to give many stars as we start habituation. We then begin to fade the reward by not rewarding as often. During the second clinical session, we find that the production of the [k] in the words is slipping. We have moved too fast. So we back up and go to a heavier reward schedule. This will solve the problem. We are not faced with the problem that the client cannot make the sound in the word. We are dealing with the "automaticity" of the production. It has not been firmly established yet. When the client is attending carefully to the production, it is correct; but as the client attends to other things, the production slips. Back to the drawing board.

Role Shifting: Talking Situations and Objects

Example 1. Our client is a 55-year-old male who, as a result of a cerebrovascular accident (CVA), is aphasic. We are seeing him in a nursing home. He is now able to communicate quite adequately except in talking situations where he becomes emotional. When this occurs, he cannot use the methods we have taught him to recall the names of things. This creates problems in the dining room of the nursing home since he is unable to order his food from the menu.

This S– situation must be dealt with not only for the emotional state of the client but also to eliminate the problem in the dining room.

We would address this problem by getting a menu from the dining room and doing some role playing in the clinic room. In that we and the clinic room are both S+, the probability that the client can successfully "order" from the menu is quite high. We first sit with the client and decide on what he would like to order from the menu. The "order" is rehearsed with the client so he is familiar with what he is going to say. We then seat the client at a table in the clinic room and walk up to him as the waiter would do in the dining room. We hand him the menu and ask for his order. This arrangement is worked through until he is secure in ordering from us. We then bring in another person and repeat the situation until he can order from this person. His confidence in ordering from the menu is strengthened and this reduces the amount of anxiety associated with ordering in the dining room.

Example 2. We are working with a 35-year-old male who stutters. His job calls for him to do a great deal of dictating, but he finds that when he picks up the microphone to dictate, his level of anxiety increases to the point where he cannot use the new speech behaviors we have taught him. The dictating equipment plays a strong S– role which we need to deal with in the clinical environment. We do not have a dictating machine available so we ask the client to bring the microphone with him when he comes in for therapy

We start our role shift of the dictating machine by having the client dictate a letter while looking at the microphone which is placed on the table directly in front of him. When he can do this while using the new speech behaviors we have taught him, we have him dictate a letter while holding the microphone in his hand at his side. The next step is dictating while holding the microphone in his hand which is resting on the arm of the chair. The situation is then repeated with the microphone held to the side of the face. Finally, we have the client dictate with the microphone held directly in front of his mouth. We have not directly worked on the dictating machine but we have reduced the S– role of the microphone and this should increase the probability that the client will be able to use the new speech behaviors while dictating in the office. We might also suggest to the client that he not look at the dictating machine while dictating. If he looks only at the microphone he will be better able to use his new speech behaviors since the microphone is no longer an S–.

PLANNING AND PROBLEM SOLVING

The following clinical situations will present some problems for you to resolve. Think these through carefully, remembering what stage of therapy we are in. Make notes of your methods of dealing with the situations and then turn to Appendix C for my discussion of the clinical situations. Again, there are many ways of dealing with clinical problems and your solution may actually be better than mine (heaven forbid).

Situation A

You have a 50-year-old male aphasic client. You have established a very basic vocabulary. However, you find that when you remove the gestural guidance prompt for the water, the client will not produce it. You now have a situation where the sequence of events is the prompt, the response, and the reward. You do not want to remove the reward at this time since you want to reward the spontaneous production of the word. How would you wean the client from the prompt?

Situation B

Your client is a 13-year-old male with cerebral palsy. You have been working on the [g] sound using a token economy. As you begin to reward every other sound production, the sound begins to deteriorate. When you go back to a constant reward schedule, the sound is stable but as soon as you move from the 1:1 ratio to a 2:1 ratio, the sound production falters. How can you remove the tokens while maintaining the correct production of the sound?

Situation C

Your 15-year-old male client came to you with a pitch problem. You have succeeded in lowering the pitch in the clinic room but the client tells you that he is afraid to use the new pitch with his peers since it is so different. He also reports that he is so tense when he is with his peers, that he cannot even produce the new pitch. It is your decision that this situation should be at least partially dealt with in the clinical environment. How would you do this?

Chapter 6

Synopsis

The new behavior is stable and habituated in the clinical environment but must now be transferred to other environments. The generalization process is a complex one and often the most difficult phase of therapy. It is in this phase of therapy that we will extend the clinical process and the CIM to our client's external environments. If we have significant others available who will work with us, we must train them to assist us and teach them how to use their interactions with the client in a home program. If no significant others are available, we must compensate for this. All of these issues are discussed in this chapter.

Chapter 6

Generalizing the New Behavior

ANTECEDENT AND CONTINGENT EVENTS IN THE CIM

We are now at that point in the clinical process where the new behavior is habituated in the clinical environment and our clinical task shifts to the transfer, or generalization, of the new behavior to other environments. We most often refer to this part of treatment as "carry-over." In my experience, this is the most difficult part of a treatment program. I have also found that this is the most challenging and time consuming part of treatment. I may have spent 4 weeks of therapy creating and habituating the new behavior in the clinical environment, and then I must spend another 12 or more weeks establishing and habituating the behavior in the client's external environments.

Because we cannot actually be with our clients in the external environments, we must depend on other factors to get the behavior to occur outside the clinic room. With many clinicians, the only factor that they appear to depend on is the habit strength of the new behavior. They feel that if the new speech habit is strong enough the new behavior will occur spontaneously in other environments. This process may succeed but, unfortunately, it is a slow and unpredictable process, particularly with younger clients who do not have approach motivation to change their speech behaviors. If a client comes to us because he wants to change his communicative behaviors, we have a built-in factor of approach motivation. But what about those clients who are sent to us? We were able to create artificial approach motivation and/or avoidance motivation for these clients within the clinical environment, but we are now faced with creating approach motivation and/or avoidance motivation to generalize the behavior to external environments. The difficulty of this task is dependent on our influence on the significant others in those environments as well as their availability and/or interest in our treatment. In order to increase the efficiency of the program to generalize the new behavior to environments other than the clinic room, we need a more specific program which, if possible, should include the client's significant others. We develop such a program in the remainder of the chapter.

As we now shift the focus of our treatment to environments other than the clinic room, the contingent events continue to be important but we will concentrate on the antecedent events, that is, the stimuli which have assumed specific roles in the client's life (conditioned stimuli). These stimuli include the significant others in the client's life, talking situations the client experiences, and objects the client associates with communication. We must recognize that the client has already established talking habits in response to these stimuli. The roles of the stimuli cue specific speech behaviors. The client has talked "incorrectly" to the significant others in his life for a lengthy period of time. The significant others have either rewarded his incorrect speech by listening to him and responding to him or penalized his speech by criticizing him. In this way the significant others assumed either the S+ or S- role for the incorrect speech.

The talking situations may have also assumed stimulus roles. If a client has talked incorrectly in the home for an extended period of time, the home can become either an S+ or an S-, depending on the response he receives for his speech in this environment. If he has talked incorrectly in the home for several years and has been rewarded for it, the home environment assumes the S+ role for the incorrect speech and cues it to occur. Talking situations often assume negative stimulus roles (S-) particularly for the client who stutters. If the client is penalized for his stuttering when talking in front of a class then this speaking situation becomes an S-, cuing the client that if he talks in front of a group he will be penalized.

Objects in the client's life such as the telephone and other objects associated with communication may have also assumed a stimulus role. If they have assumed a role of S+ for the incorrect behavior, this could create problems for us as we attempt to discourage the use of the incorrect behavior. In other instances, the objects might have the role of S-, causing negative emotions that prevent the new behavior from occurring. These stimulus roles are an important factor that must be considered as we attempt to generalize the new behavior.

Stimulus manipulation was an important part of the previous steps in the clinical process. In this step it is our main clinical tool. We have shifted the roles of the significant others in previous steps and even dealt with some talking situations and objects in the habituation step. We are now going to devote all of our attention to this clinical tool. The new behavior is now occurring on a predictable basis but it is not occurring with all of the appropriate stimuli. It is too restricted. We must generalize it so that it occurs when outside stimuli are present, not just in the clinical setting.

The clinical tasks of the clinician change drastically in this step of therapy. The behavior is occurring naturally in the clinical environment so clinical rewards and penalties are no longer necessary. The clinical tasks are now to "orchestrate" the client's external environments so that he receives rewards for the correct speech behavior and penalties for the incorrect behavior in these environments. Our "orchestration" will be accomplished through stimulus manipulation. The degree to which we can use the methods of manipulation will depend on the availability and cooperation we receive from the significant others in the external environments. Not only must the clinician carefully orchestrate the environments, she must monitor them carefully so that environmental adjustments can be made if necessary.

STIMULUS MANIPULATION

As we discuss the various methods of stimulus manipulation we will change the order of presentation from previous chapters. The reason for this is that we now have different clinical tasks and the order of importance has changed.

Increase the Number of Stimuli

Our clinical goal in this step in treatment is to increase the number of S+ which cue the new speech behavior to occur. Thus far in therapy the client has had only two S+, the clinician and the clinical environment. Where are we going to find the stimuli to add to the stimuli in the client's external environments? We are going to take S− and S0 and change them to S+. We started shifting the roles of other stimuli in the habituation step but now this becomes our main clinical task.

Role shift: Significant others. We have been shifting the roles of the significant others as we progressed through our treatment. We are now at that stage where the significant others follow the pattern of the clinician in the habituation phase. In essense, the significant others are first habituating the new behavior in their environment and then generalizing it to still other environments. Early in the generalization of the new behavior, the significant others are very strong S+, rewarding every occurrence of the new behavior. These are the strongest and most stable S+ we are going to have in the external environment so we must shift them carefully and make certain that the S+ roles are maintained in the early stages of generalizing the behavior. We will shift them again later after the behavior is stable in the external environment, but for now, the stronger the better. This shift is seen in Figure 10.

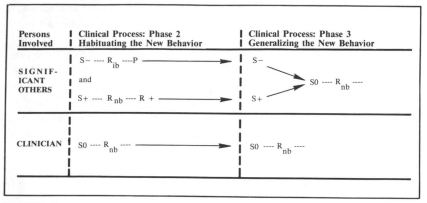

FIGURE 10
Stimulus Role Shift Model—Clinical Process: Phase 3. When the treatment program moves into Phase 3, the significant others gradually shift their stimulus roles from S+ and S– to that of S0, testing the habituation of the new behavior in the external environment by removing the reward. In that the new behavior remains stable in the clinical environment, the clinician maintains her S0 role.

Role shift: Talking situations and objects. We need to assess the talking situations and objects in our client's external environment in order to determine if any of them have an S– role. This is particularly true for those clients who stutter, but it is also a consideration with any client where negative emotions might interfere with the performance of the new behavior. When we discover talking situations or objects which have an S– role, we want to try to shift them to an S+ by associating them with rewards. If we cannot shift them to an S+ we want to at least attempt to neutralize their influence on the occurrence of the new behavior. We can shift them to an S0 by removing the penalty. But, manipulating the contingent event associated with a talking situation or an object is much more difficult than working with significant others. We do not have the same degree of control over these stimuli that we have with the significant others. In order to make this shift we have to use some other stimulus manipulation techniques.

As we discuss these techniques, let us not forget that the new behavior is occurring in the clinical environment. We are not discussing the performance of a new behavior for the client; rather, the performance of a newly *acquired* behavior in a variety of situations outside the clinical environment. If we are attempting to get the new behavior to occur in a talking situation which has an S– role, we may have to use gradual introduction of the stimuli. We are using the same procedures except that we do not have direct control over the situation since it is occurring in another environment. We must now depend on the significant others to arrange the situation so that there is a gradual buildup of the "stress" in the situation or we must depend on the client himself to approach the talking situation or the object in steps. We might tell the client who stutters to practice his new speech behavior on the telephone as he calls friends, and then acquaintances, and then on business calls. The client is then gradually presenting the S– object to himself.

Another technique we can use is the gradual withdrawal of the stimulus. In this instance we are talking about the significant others being the stimulus we are going to gradually withdraw. If a talking situation cannot be gradually presented, we may want the significant others to accompany the client into the situation. We now have an S+ associated with the S– situation. With the significant others accompanying the client, the probability of the new behavior occurring in the situation is greatly enhanced. The gradual withdrawal is then accomplished by having the significant others diminish their influence in the situation. For example, the significant others might actually accompany the client into a store while he deals with the clerk. The next time the situation arises the significant others wait at the next counter. They then wait at the door to the store. In this way they are gradually withdrawing their S+ influence as the client succeeds on his own.

Not all of our clients have S– situations. However, for those who do, such as stutterers and aphasics, it is crucial that the clinician orchestrate the environment so that the client succeeds in using his new speech behavior in or with these threatening talking situations or objects.

Decrease the number of stimuli. Here, we are interested in decreasing the number of S– in the client's external environment. We accomplish this as we increase the number of S+ through role shifting. However, there is an important exception to this. We are actually increasing the number of S– as we shift the roles of the significant others to S– for the incorrect behavior. This is a highly controlled role shift of the significant others. We are doing this so that we can discourage the performance of the incorrect behavior in the most important external environment, usually the home.

We use all of the stimulus manipulation techniques as we attempt to generalize the client's new behavior, but now let us go directly to the clinical process and see how this is applied.

EXTENDING THE CLINICAL PROCESS

At this stage of the game there has been a major change in the clinical process. We are no longer working within a single environment. We are now working in two general environments, the clinical environment and the external environment. The clinical activities in the two environments are very different.

The Clinical Environment

The clinician is no longer working directly with the client's speech behavior. She now has new "clients" if the significant others are involved in the clinical program. She has to teach them how to work with the client in their environment. They must get the new behavior to occur in their environment, habituate it there, and then generalize it to other environments. Their role in all of this is very similar to the role of the clinician as we have progressed through the clinical process to this point in therapy. Therapy is now done through the significant others and the clinician becomes more of an orchestrator and consultant than a clinician. She instructs the significant others following the same guidelines (the CIM) she used when teaching the client his new speech behavior. She is going to provide modeling, information, and guidance for the significant others and, at the same time, monitor their attention to the learning process and evaluate how much they have learned. She will reward and penalize them to create approach motivation and/or avoidance motivation to carry on the home program. Essentially, she is providing the significant others with a "crash course" in therapy. She will set up the programs in the external environment, but the significant others are charged with implementing them.

The clinical sessions at this point in therapy are divided between the clinician's monitoring of the speech behaviors of the client and her monitoring of the significant others' program through their reports, either verbal or written. She will have to be extremely careful about the types and amounts of rewards and penalties the significant others are administering. She must also monitor the gradual fading of the rewards through changing the reward schedule. It is a tough job but there does not seem to be any easy way to get new speech behaviors to generalize.

Speaking of tough jobs, what does the clinician do if she has no significant others to assist with the generalization of the new behavior? In this situation the clinician must either find other people in the client's external environment who will help with the generalization process or she will have to figure out ways she can do it. It is very difficult to find other people to assist us. If we turn to teachers in the schools we must realize that they have their own teaching to do and they are extremely busy with their own problems. The same holds true in other environments such as nursing homes or hospitals. These other people will often provide what help they can but it is quite limited since they have their own tasks to perform. All of this planning, bargaining, plotting, and manipulating goes on in the clinical environment. This is the clinician's job at this point in therapy. Now let us consider the fruits of this labor. How are things planned for the external environment?

The External Environment

We need to be more specific about the external environment(s) in this discussion. For most of our clients, the external environment we are working with is the home environment. This is where we want the new behavior to occur and from there, we hope, it will generalize to all of the other environments of the client. It is impossible for us to work directly with each of the client's environments. As the new speech behavior becomes more stable and more habituated, it will generalize to many environments without direct assistance. Early in the generalization of the new behavior we must provide as much assistance and support as possible.

There are four unique circumstances that we must deal with as we generalize the new behavior. We have clients who are highly motivated to change their behavior and we have clients who have no motivation to change their behavior. There are significant others who cooperate with us and assist in the generalization of the new behavior as well as absent or disinterested significant others who provide no assistance. (There are even significant others who work against us, a problem discussed in Chapter 8.) We need to discuss the generalization procedure in all four situations. We start with the ideal situation and save the worst for last. By arranging the discussion this way, we may be able to pick up some helpful hints in the easier situations which will help us with the more difficult situations.

Motivated client: Assistance from significant others. The therapy in the external environment consists of three phases. We must first of all get the new behavior to occur in the environment, then habituate it in that environment, and finally generalize it to other environments.

Getting the new behavior to occur. In the previous step in therapy we shifted the roles of the significant others to S+ for the new behavior and S- for the old behavior. We should have the behavior occurring in the external environment if the significant others are rewarding its occurrences and the client has approach motivation to change his behavior. If not, we may have to work with the client with the significant others present in the clinical setting. When the new behavior occurs for us, we have the significant others give the reward. This is a more direct way of creating their new S+ role. The S+ role is important with this type of client as a supplement to the client's own motivation. The S- role is of lesser importance since the client already has approach motivation. If the approach motivation lags as generalization progresses, we can still turn to avoidance motivation, but it may not need to be used.

We must monitor the significant others carefully in such a home program. All they know about the clinical process is what we have taught them. If things are so simple that you can train significant others completely in a couple of hours, why does it take so many years to train a competent speech clinician? Keep in mind that the significant others have no deep insights into why they are doing what they are doing. They are following your instructions.

If the new behavior is not stable in the external environment, the significant others may have to do some modeling. This can be easily explained to the significant others in terms of having them show the client how the new behavior should be performed. At the most, this should be a short-term arrangement. The behavior has not been forgotten. It is just that the transfer of the behavior to the external environment is too big a step for the client. Some modeling with constant rewards for performing the new behavior should rectify this situation quickly. And do not forget we have the approach motivation of the client working for us.

The most difficult task, I have found, is to get the significant others to maintain their S+ and S- roles long enough for the new behavior to generalize. They tend to feel that when the new behavior has occurred and been rewarded several times this is sufficient. I mention this problem here because I have had difficulty with some significant others maintaining their roles even during this first phase of the home program. Giving the significant others heavy doses of reward for maintaining their roles seems to do the trick.

Habituating the new behavior. Habituation is accomplished just as we did it in the clinical environment. We adjust the ratio of rewards so that the significant others gradually shift their roles again. We slowly withdraw the S+ and S- roles as the behavior establishes itself in the new environment. Again, we are testing habituation. If the new behavior begins to falter, the significant others must increase the amount of reward associated with it. As mentioned earlier, it is not uncommon for the significant others to tend to rush the withdrawal of rewards. They need to recognize that even though a behavior might be quite stable in their environment, it might be just getting established in other environments. It is much better to extend the reward system beyond its useful time than to terminate it before the behavior is stabilized. The significant others must be carefully monitored in order to maintain the gradual withdrawal of the reward.

Generalizing the new behavior. In most instances, once the new behavior is habituated in the significant others' environment it will naturally generalize to the client's other environments. However, in some cases the client's new behavior occurs in the significant others' environment but does not occur in other environments. These clients need a cue or prompt to help them remember to produce the new behavior when there are no S+ or S- in the environment. We must remember that in the other environments there may be talking situations and objects that have assumed an S- role. Other people, such as authority figures, may have also assumed such a role. This is where gradual presentation and gradual withdrawal of the stimuli come in handy.

As the client starts to generalize his new behavior to other environments, the significant others can use "reminders" to help the client. A reminder is anything unusual which, when noticed, reminds a person to do something. An example will make the idea clear. One client would turn over a chair in the middle of the kitchen when he wanted to remember something important. He would then come down to the kitchen in the morning and wonder why there was a chair upside down in the middle of the floor. This would remind him that he did it in order to remember to do something important like make a telephone call. This worked very well for him until he came down to the kitchen in the middle of the night for a snack and fell over the chair in the dark. He broke the chair and his leg. He decided to change his reminder to a slipper on the bathroom counter.

Here is a list of some reminders I have taught significant others to use to help clients remember to produce the new behavior:

1. A Band-Aid on a finger.
2. A string around a finger.
3. Wearing the watch on the "wrong" wrist.
4. A small adhesive "dot" on the side of the lens of the glasses.
5. Carrying an unusual object in a trousers' pocket.
6. Wearing a ring on the "wrong" finger.
7. Wearing a bracelet on the "wrong" wrist.
8. A ball and chain on the ankle.

This should give you an idea of what I use as reminders. Each of these things will last for only a short time. As soon as the client becomes accustomed to the reminder, it no longer helps. We must change these often in order for them to provide the cue or prompt for the client.

We can also use verbal reports by the client to both us and the significant others as to how well he is able to use the new speech behavior in other environments. However, there is a better way to achieve this information than to rely on the client's memory. We can have the client keep a log book of his talking situations where he is practicing his new speech behavior in other environments. The client should share his log book with us and the significant others. In that the log book forms the core of our work with clients when there are no significant others to work with us, we discuss the use of the log book in detail in the following section. However, remember that the log book can be used effectively with clients where the significant others are working with us.

Motivated client: No assistance from significant others. When we are sometimes faced with a situation where the significant others are either not available or not interested in assisting with the therapy program, our first step is to try to arrange to have other people in the client's external environment assist us in generalization. As we discussed earlier, this poses a problem in terms of coordinating their efforts and making sure they are consistent in their rewards and penalties. It is also a problem finding another person who has, or will take, the time to help us. We should try to find people who can assume S+ and S– roles.

Our first clinical task in generalizing the behavior is to select some external environment where we can concentrate our efforts. This might well be that environment where we are able to find other people who would work with us. If we cannot get assistance we must work with the client to determine an appropriate environment. With a motivated client this is not a difficult task. We might decide on a work environment with an adult client or a particular classroom environment with a younger client. In any event, we should focus our efforts on a specific environment rather than use a "shotgun" approach, that is, working with all of the client's environments at the same time.

Once we have decided on the environment where the client is going to start using the new behavior, we must figure out some way of getting the client to use the new behavior, and a method of reporting his success or failure to us. This is vital information since, if the client is failing in his attempts to use the new behavior, we must change our approach so that he can succeed. If we have no significant others to work with us we cannot set up a structured program as we did in the previous section. We will follow the same general procedures, but, since we have so little control over the external environments, we will need to make adjustments as we go along.

Log book. My most successful approach to this clinical situation has been with the speech "log book." I carefully explain to the client that the log book is for recording his speech *practice* and his speech *game* situations. Practice occurs when the client is concentrating on *how* he is talking rather than on *what* he is talking about. During these situations, the client is making a very special effort to have the new speech behavior occur. It might even be necessary for some clients to memorize what they are going to say so that, when the situation does occur, they can concentrate on *how* they are talking. Let us think of this in terms of the client's attention being directed 75% toward *how* he is talking and 25% on *what* he is talking about. A game is talking, such as in a conversation, while attending 75% to *what* is being said and only 25% to *how* it is being said.

I explain the difference between practice and games to the client by drawing an analogy with learning to play tennis. The coach provides modeling, guidance, and information regarding how to hold the racket, how to serve the ball, and how to perform the backhand. The coach then has the player practice each procedure independently. For the serve, the player stands at the line and serves 40 balls to the other side of the court. There is no return of the ball, just practice of the serve. For the backhand, the coach hits balls to the player in such a way that the player can practice returning the ball with the backhand. After several weeks of practice of the various moves in tennis, the player enters a game with another person. He will not be practicing during the game, he will be testing to see how well he has learned through his practice. He will find out in the game how much more he needs to practice and on what moves.

The log book is primarily for recording the practice of the new speech behavior in the external environment. There may be four or five practice sessions each day. However, each practice session is quite short since the client will find it very difficult to concentrate on *how* he is talking for an extended period of time. As the behavior becomes more stable in the external environments the practice sessions can last longer. At that time, the client can also include reports on games, for example, conversations where he attempted to use the new behavior.

The size of the log book is also an important item. It should be small enough to carry in a pocket since I want the client to carry it with him at all times. The only times that the client may be without the log book are in the shower and when sleeping. It cannot function to remind him to practice his new speech behaviors, or to record the success of the practice, if it is at home on a table. I have the client purchase a small spiral notebook with the spiral along the edge rather than along the top. You may not consider this important but I can never tell the front from the back if the spiral is on top. I never know which way to turn the pages. You may have to learn this the hard way, just as I did.

I have the clients enter very specific information for each practice session. First I have them write down enough information about the practice so that they can remember it when we discuss it. This is usually just a couple of words to remind the clients what the situation was. Depending on the client, I then have them rate their stress as they go into the practice situation. Talking situations vary in terms of the amount of stress. Speaking to a peer may be easier for the client than speaking to a group of peers, which might be easier than speaking to a large group of authority figures. As the client is put under more stress, the probability that he will be able to use his new speaking behavior correctly is diminished. Thus, if we can have the client record the amount of stress he is experiencing when he enters a practice situation, we can adjust our expectations. My clients rate their stress on a 5-point scale where a (1) situation is the easiest and a (5) situation is the most stressful. I expect a better performance in a (1) or (2) situation than I do in a (4) or (5) situation. It also helps the client understand why he may perform his new behavior better in one situation than in another.

The client enters the first two items in the log book before he goes into the practice situation. He has identified the situation and rated the degree of stress of the situation. He now practices his new speech behavior. Upon completion of the practice I have the client rate his degree of stress again using the same 5-point scale. I have found that this is very important. If the client has had a very successful practice and was able to use the new speech behavior, the degree of stress in the situation will reduce. The client might go into a practice situation he rated a (4) but, after a very successful practice, the stress is reduced and the client now rates the situation a (3). He is gaining self-confidence in using the new behavior. This is a vital component in the treatment of the aphasic, the stutterer, and other clients where there is emotional involvement in the disorder.

The next bit of information I need from the client is some sort of indication of how well he was able to use the new behavior. The easiest thing I have found is a simple grading system; "A" for perfect use to an "E" for inability to use it. Yes, it is subjective, but at least it is some sort of indication of what is going on when the client is working on his own. In using the grading system I must train the client to grade his speech. I compare his grade with my own and we adjust his level of expectancy to mine. Essentially, I am calibrating the client to be a good judge of his speech so that I can keep track of his success in generalizing his speech behavior.

The analysis of the log book in the therapy session is rather detailed. Let us examine an example of three situations a client might bring in and how they would be analyzed for him.

LOG BOOK

Situation 1	Situation 2	Situation 3
1. lunch	1. nurse	1. phone
2. 4	2. 3	2. 4
3. 2	3. 3	3. 3
4. B+	4. B	4. B–

This client is an adult aphasic who is in a nursing home and this is the environment we have decided to focus on. We have worked on some of these talking situations and objects while we were in the habituation phase of therapy. His log book reports that he practiced his new speech behavior (recalling the names of objects) in three situations. He ordered his lunch, talked to the nurse, and made a telephone call to his family. He indicated that there was a lot of stress in the practice situations with ordering lunch and telephoning being (4) situations. These ratings indicate that the client expected to have a great deal of difficulty in the talking situations. But the ratings he made after the practice indicated that he was quite successful and lost some of the fear of the talking situations and the object. We had rehearsed ordering lunch and he did a good job. His stress was reduced from a (4) to a (2). We also worked on the telephone and this situation also showed a reduction in stress from a (4) to a (3). The only situation that did not result in reduced stress was talking to the nurse, but we had not rehearsed this. Still, the practice was very successful. He reported that his speech was at a Grade "B" level. The lowest grade he gave himself was the "B–" on the telephone.

The degree of success is reviewed with the client on a highly cognitive level. His success is strongly rewarded through verbal praise and pointing out carefully how well he did in using his new speech. The client's log book is carefully reviewed in each therapy session with a heavy emphasis on rewarding him for his success. As the client gains confidence, the first rating of stress (Item Number 2) reduces. Ordering lunch reduces from a (4), to a (3), to a (2), and so on. It eventually reaches a point where the expectation of stress lowers to the point where it matches the actual stress experienced. This is a strong indication that some significant cognitive changes are taking place.

At the same time, the grades for speech improve. I compare the grades with the second rating of stress (Item Number 3). If the client has collected 35 practice situations in a week, I list all of the grades for each level of stress.

As the client practices the new behavior in the environment and gains confidence, the grades improve. My analysis might look like this:

(5)   D, D, D+

(4)   D+, C–, C, C+, C+

(3)   C–, C, C, C+, C+, B, B

(2)   C, C, C+, C, C+, B, B–, B, B+

(1)   B–, B, B–, B, B, B+, B+, A–, B+, A–, A

Your records may not look this good, but then, as the author, I can stretch reality a bit. The point is that the grades will improve over time. As I analyzed the (2) situations, for example, I might point out to the client that the week started with grades of "C" for the new speech behavior but that after nine practices during the week, he had raised the grade up to a "B+." I would give a lot of verbal praise for raising the grade that much in only one week.

We must remember that in this clinical situation where we have a motivated client but no significant other involvement, the only person who is actively supporting the client is us. We are his one and only support system. If we are trying to increase the number of S+ to encourage the new behavior to occur, let us look to the log book. First of all, it serves as a reminder for the client to perform his behavior. It also results in rewards from me when we review and analyze it. Through this association with me and my rewards, the log book becomes a very strong S+. It is almost an extension of me into the client's external environment, reminding the client to perform his practice and cuing the new behavior to occur.

When we had cooperation from the significant others we had both an S+ and S–. The log book also assumes the role of S–. In fact, it assumes two S– roles. First of all, it serves as an S– cuing the incorrect behavior not to occur since there may be some penalty associated with this when I review the report, although I do keep penalty at a minimum unless I must use the client's avoidance motivation. Our client in this example has high approach motivation so there will be little need to turn to avoidance motivation. This does not mean that we abandon penalty, we only use less of it.

The second S– role the log book assumes concerns filling a quota of practice sessions. If the client is required to report four practice sessions per day, there is penalty if less than the quota is handed in. In this S– role, the log book cues the client to do his practice sessions in order to avoid my penalizing him. How much "fudging" do I get? Some, definitely, but usually not with a highly motivated client. Usually the client just says that he did not have the time to collect all of the practice sessions requested. If I have requested four per day but the client is consistently coming up one or two short, I negotiate with the client. I adjust the number required to the number of sessions he has been able to do in the past. Now, there are no excuses. He has set the quota.

The log book is as helpful in therapy as the clinician wants it to be. The assistance the clinician receives from the log book depends on the clarity of the data the client is to enter into the log book; the frequency and depth of analysis of the data by the clinician and the client; and the appropriateness, frequency, and consistency of the rewards and penalties associated with the log book reports. When used to its fullest extent, the log book is the strongest tool the speech clinician has for generalizing new speech behaviors. It is even stronger than most programs where the significant others are giving assistance. But, you say, what do you do for children? I have used the log book with children as young as 5 years of age. As long as they can count and write from 1 to 5 and from "A" to "E," I can adjust the log book to them. It just takes some imagination.

Now let us move into those clinical situations where we are working with clients who are not motivated to work on their speech.

Unmotivated client: Assistance from the significant others. This clinical program is going to be quite similar to the first situation where we had a client with approach motivation and cooperation from the significant others. With the unmotivated client we had to create artificial approach motivation in the clinical environment through the use of carefully selected rewards. We also had to use the client's avoidance motivation to avoid our penalties. This works quite effectively in the clinical environment since we have direct control over the clinical environment. However, now we have to create the same artificial approach motivation and avoidance motivation in the external environment. Since the client is not motivated to work on his speech, we must give him approach motivation to achieve the reward and avoidance motivation to avoid the penalty from the significant others.

We will follow the same home program that we used for the client who has approach motivation. However, we are now totally dependent on the rewards and penalties from the significant others for the client's approach motivation and avoidance motivation. We must be extremely careful in our instructions to the significant others. They will need more insight into what they are doing and why they are doing it. The rewards and penalties must be carefully selected. The token economy is particularly well adapted to this type of situation, for most younger clients fall into this unmotivated classification. They do not see the importance of changing their speech. The significant others must provide the approach motivation and avoidance motivation in the home environment through rewards and penalties.

Getting the new behavior to occur. There are some changes in emphasis in the program with the unmotivated client. We have to be very careful in establishing the significant others as S+ and S-. This is our only means of creating approach motivation and avoidance motivation with this client. We should not rush this step. Make certain that the new S+ and S– roles are firmly established before starting the generalization program in the significant others' environment.

We will also need to monitor the home program more carefully here. We are not to the stage of maintaining the client's approach motivation and avoidance motivation since we must first of all create them. We have given special training to the significant others so their reports to us will be a bit more detailed than in other situations. This detailed information allows us to make corrections when needed both in creating and maintaining the client's approach motivation and avoidance motivation.

There may, indeed, be more need for modeling of behaviors by the significant others with this type of client. They should understand what modeling is and why it is used. As the behavior becomes more stable in the significant others' environment, the amount of modeling can be reduced but it should not be withdrawn too soon or too quickly. This is where our monitoring comes in. The reports from the significant others are very important.

In all probability the therapy with the unmotivated client will proceed slower than with the motivated client. For this reason, the significant others will have to maintain their S+ and S– roles for an extended period of time. I mentioned that I had difficulty in getting the significant others to maintain their roles with motivated clients. It is even more difficult with unmotivated clients since progress in generalization is slower. Do not forget to reward the significant others for all of the assistance they are giving you. This is a good way to maintain their roles. And, if you are clever enough, you can also work in some penalty.

Habituating the new behavior. There is really no change in procedure from that of the motivated client. I would only caution that the process cannot be rushed. It is slower than with motivated clients but we must accept this and direct the significant others accordingly. We are faced with an interesting problem here. How do we determine if our generalization is going too slowly or if we are moving too fast? As in love and war, there are no rules. This is a professional judgment on our part and comes with experience. But, if a clinician takes 2 years to generalize a sound into a client's external environment, this is hard to justify. Perhaps you can use as a guideline the old saying, "Let your conscience be your guide."

Generalizing the new behavior. The most radical change in this phase of generalization will be in the use of reminders. Since the client is unmotivated, the reminders have little, if any, effect. This is true since there is no specific reward associated with the reminder. How can we correct the situation? We can start by shifting to the log book with a strong reward program. Even though the client is not interested in working on his speech we provide him with approach motivation to achieve the reward. We use the log book to keep track of how many or much reward he receives. If he has approach motivation to achieve the reward we can use his avoidance motivation to avoid losing the reward. Let us not forget that the significant others are cooperating with us in our therapy. It is important that we have the client share the log book with the significant others so they can provide support through rewards.

We are also going to have to provide some direct assistance to this client as we attempt to generalize the new behavior to other environments, including talking situations and objects. Since the significant others are cooperating with us and they have assumed the S+ role, it is important that they assist the client in transferring the behavior outside the significant others' environment. They can use gradual presentation and gradual withdrawal of the stimuli as an aid here.

This step in generalizing the behavior with this type of client is exceptionally difficult since neither the clinician nor the significant others have direct control over the other environments. There needs to be careful monitoring of the significant others' program, and they need all of the guidance that the clinician can give them. After all, they are doing the clinician's work. The least we can do is help them.

Unmotivated client: No assistance from significant others. Now we have reached the most difficult of all clinical tasks. We were able to deal with this client in the clinical environment since we had direct control over the rewards and penalties. We created approach motivation and avoidance motivation in the clinic room but now we must transfer the behavior to other environments. Who can we turn to for help? We might try to find people in the client's external environments who would be willing to help but this is extremely limited in terms of its effectiveness. We have the same problems of consistency and coordination. But keep in mind that we have a client who is not interested in changing his speech.

The only things we have that we can use are rewards and penalties. We have assumed the S+ and S– roles but it is very difficult to get other people to establish these roles. They may not be in contact with the client often enough or long enough to establish the roles. Also, they may not be consistent enough for the role to "take." This does not mean that we should not try to get other people to assume the S+ and S– roles. With this type of client we need all the help we can get. We should also recognize that it is going to be difficult to establish and to maintain the behavior.

The most important thing that we must do is maintain the approach motivation and avoidance motivation that we have established with the client in the clinic room. The rewards and penalties had to be appropriate or we could not have created the approach motivation and avoidance motivation in the client.

We now apply these as the client takes the new behavior outside. What is the best way to do this? I have found that the best tool I have available is the log book. I can manipulate the log book so that it becomes an S+ and an S− in the external environments. As long as the rewards and penalties are appropriate, the log book will assist in the generalization of the new speech behavior.

With younger clients, where the log book cannot be used, the clinician must devise some other way for the client to report on outside practice so that there can be a reward. We have to maintain the approach motivation and avoidance motivation we created in the clinic room and we cannot stop rewarding and penalizing when the client is generalizing the behavior to other environments. If a log book is not practical, perhaps a reward book could be used. We must devise something so that the client can keep track of how well he is doing.

Is it best to establish a single external environment where the client will be expected to perform the new speech behavior? Yes. This is important so that the client can initially direct his efforts to a single environment and so that the clinician can plan the generalization program in this restricted environment. As the new behavior stabilizes in this environment, other environments (including talking situations and objects) can be added to the practice situations in the log book. We must make the process simple enough so that we can exert as much control as possible over the external environment and yet not so simple that the client is not challenged.

Can we try to establish approach motivation and avoidance motivation in this client through a cognitive approach? It certainly will not hurt to try. As we said earlier, we can use all of the assistance we can find. If the client is an adult we can approach him either intellectually or emotionally. We can set forth facts and other data or we can make an emotional appeal. There is no denying that attitudes, emotions, feelings, and other such factors influence therapy. They must be dealt with when they are interfering with clinical progress. This aspect of therapy is discussed in detail in Chapter 8.

You will note that this is the shortest discussion of the four clinical situations, even though it is the most difficult. The reason for this is the limited resources we have when faced with this situation. But, as I said earlier in the chapter, perhaps you have gained some insights into how to handle this situation as we discussed the easier ones. In most instances, we cannot plan ahead for this clinical situation, we must improvise as we go along. I hope that the strategies discussed earlier in the chapter will help you when you find yourself with an unmotivated client and no significant others to help you generalize the new behavior.

Before we move on to our discussion of clinical examples of generalizing the new behavior to other environments you might wish to reexamine Figure 6 in Chapter 2. We have now completed the clinical process and the figure will now be more meaningful to you. When it was first presented it indicated where we were going in our discussion. It now represents where we have been and should serve as a quick reference and overview of the clinical process and the CIM.

CLINICAL EXAMPLES

Motivated Client: Assistance from Significant Others

This client is a 37-year-old male. He is a physician who has recently relocated from South America to the United States. In addition to his private medical practice, he is a lecturer at a university medical school. Unfortunately, his foreign accent is so pronounced that his students, as well as his patients, have difficulty understanding him. His wife does not have any accent, having been born and raised in the United States. Our client has avoidance motivation to change his accent because of the negative effect it is having on both his practice and his position at the university. We have focused our clinical efforts on modification of certain vowels which are either distorted or used incorrectly. He is able to use the vowels correctly in the clinical environment where there are enough S+ to cue their occurrence. However, in other environments, the original vowel habit pattern persists.

We discuss the problem of generalization with the client and his wife and the wife volunteers to work on the speech in the home environment. With our client's consent, we set up a home program in order to shift the wife's role from that of an S0 to an S+. Since we are working with a highly motivated, intelligent adult we do not have to turn to a token economy. Our task is to maintain the client's motivation by providing him with a sufficient reward for successful modification of his accent. We instruct the client and his wife to set up a regular time each evening when the client can tell his wife about his activities during the day. We suggest that the talking period be held at a regular time and to limit it to 10 minutes. During the discussion the client is instructed to use the new speech behaviors he has perfected in the clinical environment. Furthermore, we instruct the wife to reward his successful efforts. She is cautioned not to interrupt him in order to reward him, but to interject her rewards at the end of phrases or thought units. Her reward consists of verbal praise.

If the client uses a vowel incorrectly during the phrase or thought unit, the wife is to make note of the particular word and have the client repeat it correctly at the end of the phrase. If there is any difficulty in saying the word correctly, we instruct the wife to say it for him, providing him with a model. By using this method the wife penalizes the client for his mistakes by having him repeat the incorrect words. This has the effect of creating the S- role for the wife. We do not encounter any difficulty with this arrangement with this client because of his high degree of avoidance motivation.

The reward and penalty schedule in the home gradually changes as the client becomes more proficient at using the vowels correctly in this environment. We must remember that this is not a new behavior that the client is introducing into the home. He has the behavior in the clinical environment and we are simply extending it to the home. Eventually, the wife will not have to provide rewards or penalties as the incorrect speech behaviors disappear and are replaced by the habituated correct behaviors.

Now, we might have to extend our generalization program into our client's work environment. This would be very difficult in the medical practice, but our client's lectures at the medical school give us an opportunity. We ask the wife if she would be able to sit in on some of her husband's lectures. In that she is both an S+ and an S-, her presence in the lecture hall should cue the new behaviors to occur and discourage the occurrence of the old behaviors. A highly motivated client such as this would not object to this type of arrangement (unless the school insisted that his wife pay tuition for attending the class).

Motivated Client: No Assistance from Significant Others

We are working with a 27-year-old female who is a singer with a rock band. She eventually developed vocal nodes from vocal abuse and went to a physician for an examination. He referred her to us to see if we could eliminate enough of the vocal abuse so that the nodes would be absorbed. We determined that the main source of vocal abuse was the hard vocal attack, not only in her singing but in her everyday speech. When in the clinical environment, she can use an easy vocal attack consistently in conversations and singing. We now need to extend this new behavior to her everyday conversations and, we hope, to her professional singing. Our problem is that she has no significant others who will work with her in changing her vocal behavior.

Our best tool in this situation is the log book. We instruct the client that we want her to practice the new vocal attack in specific talking situations in her everyday speech. However, we are going to have to make some changes in the types of information we want her to bring to us. We have her include the following information in her log book: (1) information to identify the talking situation; (2) a rating on a 1 to 5 scale of the effort used in initiating voice; (3) a grade from "A" to "E" which reflects her success in using the easy vocal attack; and (4) if she failed to use her easy vocal attack, what factors there were in the situation that prevented her from using the new vocal attack. The log book provides us with several important features in achieving generalization of the new behavior. Most important, the log book assumes both an S+ and S- role, since it is closely associated with us. We carefully review the log book during each clinical session and this association is what makes the role shift possible for the log book itself. The log book cues the new behavior to occur and discourages the occurrence of the incorrect behavior.

Second, the log book functions as a reminder. We have instructed the client to carry the book with her at all times. Its presence will then be a reminder. She may see the book in her purse but decide not to use the next talking situation for practice. But she saw the book and, through its S+ role, it cues the new behavior to occur, increasing the possibility that the easy vocal attack will occur.

Finally, when we review the log book with the client we emphasize her successful use of the new vocal behavior. We maintain a heavy reward schedule for her success in her everyday talking situations. This is very important since we are the only support system she has. She needs to have someone who is aware of and pleased with her progress outside the clinical environment. The log book is our only contact with our client's performance outside the clinical setting.

Depending on our clinical setting and the agency where we are working, we might even arrange to go out on some talking situations with the client. For example, we might take the regularly scheduled clinical meeting time and go to a store in the vicinity and have the client talk to some of the clerks in the store. This would be very helpful for the client since our presence as an S+ would influence the occurrence of the new behavior and we would also be able to provide immediate feedback in terms of the success of the situation.

We still have not dealt with our client's professional singing. We could have her use the log book during her rehearsals with the band, reporting her success in using the new vocal attack while performing. We might also consider going to one of her performances so our S+ role would have some influence on the behavior. We could also have her carry her log book with her as she is performing. These alternatives depend on too many variables to list here, but they are considerations we should make in working with this client.

Unmotivated Client: Assistance from Significant Others

Our client is a 17-year-old female stutterer. She has been in therapy for several months and has made excellent progress on her speech. When she started therapy she was not even able to say her name in a casual situation. At the beginning of therapy she was highly motivated to change her speech behaviors. She did her outside speaking assignments and kept her log book faithfully.

At this point in therapy she is able to speak in all situations, but she is not using her speech controls to the maximum. Her interest in therapy has dwindled since she no longer has a severe stuttering problem. Whereas before therapy she would have been considered a severe stutterer, she would now be judged to be a mild stutterer. When she uses her speech controls, her speech is normal and stuttering blocks do not occur. The clinical task is to create either approach motivation or avoidance motivation in order to generalize the excellent speech she can produce when she is controlling her speech. When asked if she wants to improve her speech in her external environments she says that it is very important to her since she knows how well she can speak when she controls her stuttering. However, she does not have the approach motivation or avoidance motivation to work on her speech in the external environments. She does not work on her log book or attempt to control her stuttering in her everyday speaking situations.

Her parents are very cooperative and would like to have their daughter use the controlled speech in all situations. They realize that she can speak normally when she makes the effort. We have a conference with the parents and the client and attempt to determine if a token economy can be set up. We look for something the client wants to achieve (a reward) or something the client does not want to lose (a penalty). During the conversation the subject of the client's car is brought up. The client uses the car every day and this is her major source of social interaction since there is no public transportation near her home.

The client already has the approach motivation to drive the car. We can then use this source of approach motivation to get her to work on her speech. We select the home environment since, through the significant others, we can control it. We then set up the following token economy. During the time the client is in the home the parents are to respond to her speech by either presenting tokens (rewards) for controlled speech or taking tokens away (penalty) for uncontrolled speech. We use both approach motivation and avoidance motivation in this economy. The client must "purchase" the use of the car each day, that is, she must have a certain number of tokens in order to use the car. To get the tokens she must use her good speech when talking in the home. The parents give her a token for good speech, not after every word, but after a certain amount of time. This is the variable interval form of intermittent reward. We are rewarding her for controlling her speech.

We are also interested in getting the client to monitor her speech more carefully so that she is aware that her speech is slipping and makes the appropriate corrections. In order to get this behavior to increase in frequency of occurrence we will have to reward her monitoring and corrections. We then tell the parents that if the client's speech slips into the stuttering pattern but the client makes a correction, bringing the speech back under control, they are to give her two tokens. Her self-monitoring and correction is an extremely important behavior so we are rewarding it even more than the controlled speech.

We now have the approach motivation to work on the speech since, if the client does not control the speech and make corrections, she does not earn the necessary number of tokens to get the car each day. But we also want to consider the consequences of the stuttering when it occurs. Since the client can produce both controlled speech and stuttering, we want to reward the controlled speech to increase its occurrence and, at the same time, penalize the stuttering to decrease the frequency of its occurrence. Our final instructions to the parents are that they should remove three tokens whenever the client uses the uncontrolled speech and fails to monitor it and make corrections. We are then penalizing not only the uncontrolled speech but also the failure to monitor and make corrections. Our client now has a great deal of avoidance motivation to avoid losing three tokens for failing to work on her speech. In order to make up for this single failure she must have three successful uses of her controlled speech.

As you can see, we are focusing both on avoidance motivation and approach motivation, with the penalty being the strongest contingent event. We are penalizing the client for failure to use the controlled speech or to monitor her speech and make the proper corrections. Our rationale is that if we penalize the uncontrolled speech, it will occur less often. What does the client use in its place? She uses controlled speech.

Unmotivated Client: No Assistance from Significant Others

We are faced with a 4-year-old male who has had his cleft palate repaired, but who still has too much nasality in his speech. This effect is also present in the production of the plosive consonants which are distorted. He was brought to us by his parents who decided that their child's speech was creating problems for the child in nursery school. Although other children were mimicking him, the child was not aware of his speech difficulties and was not bothered by the teasing of the other children.

We were able to create artificial approach motivation in the clinical environment through our reward system, a token economy with numerous rewards. We also were able to utilize the client's avoidance motivation through a penalty system where he would lose a token if nasality was present. We were successful in modifying the speech and habituating it in the clinical environment. Conferences with the parents were difficult to arrange because both parents were professionals, one an attorney and the other a physician. During the few conferences we were able to arrange, the parents reported that there was no change in the client's speech in the home or at school.

When a conference was held to arrange a program to extend the new speech behaviors into the home environment we were met with seeming cooperation from the parents. However, after the program was instituted in the home, the parents found one excuse after another as to why they were unable to carry out the home program. There was no follow-through on the part of the parents and, as a result, there was no generalization of the new behavior. Our first effort to correct this situation was to have a lengthy conference with the parents where we pointed out the need for their assistance in generalizing the behavior. Again, although they expressed an interest in following the program at home, the program was not instituted. We finally realized that there would be no cooperation from the child's parents and that we would have to approach the problem from another angle.

If the client were older we might be able to work with him on a log book or work with him on a cognitive level to create approach motivation. But we are faced with a 4-year-old. Our only good option, if we are going to follow through with this client, is to approach the nursery school teacher and see if she is willing to assist us. If she is willing to cooperate, we can set up an extension of the token economy in the school where she would reward him for eliminating the nasality from his speech. We would use a strong reward program in this instance in order to create approach motivation in the school environment. Penalty would not be used in this instance due to the lack of control we have over the school environment and the lack of professional background the teacher has in speech therapy. In order to institute such a program, we will have to meet with the teacher and identify for her the speech productions that will be rewarded and those where there is nasality and the distortion of plosive consonants where there is no reward. With careful monitoring of this program we hope that the behavior will generalize to the school and, finally, to the home.

Our other alternative is to continue working with the child in the clinical environment and trust that the new speech behavior will eventually generalize to other environments due to the strength of the behavior in the clinical situation. As I said earlier, this type of clinical situation is our most difficult challenge and it is not limited to children. Unmotivated clients with no significant others' support pose many clinical problems, and each must be dealt with in a unique fashion. There are just no simple answers to this problem.

PLANNING AND PROBLEM SOLVING

Situation A

The client in the situation is a 67-year-old widowed male who has had a laryngectomy. He is retired and living alone in an apartment complex with many other retired people. Although he has done a good job producing esophageal speech in the clinic room, he is still very depressed and fearful about the effects his condition will have on his life. You are now ready to extend the new speech behavior to other environments. What are the problems you would face here and how would you deal with them?

Situation B

Your client is a 14-year-old female with an extremely husky and low-pitched voice. She is usually mistaken for a male when on the phone and strangers react overtly when they first hear her voice. She was referred to you by her counselor in the high school. Your contact with the parents indicated that they were also concerned about the problem and they came in for several conferences during your therapy. They discuss the voice problem with their daughter at home and send you reports on any changes in the voice production at home.

You have achieved a new pitch level with the client which she can maintain in the clinical environment. At the higher pitch level, the huskiness of the voice is eliminated. However, the client does not use the new voice in any other environment. She reports that she likes the new voice but it sounds so different from her original voice that her friends look startled when she uses it. She also reports that she is extremely tense when she is about to try it outside the clinic room. The tension makes it almost impossible to produce the new voice. What problems might you face with this client and how might you deal with them in order to achieve generalization?

Situation C

This client is 65 years old and has had a stroke. He is retired and living at home with his wife. His main difficulty was in comprehending what was said to him. You have taught him strategies to assist him in comprehension and he is functioning with no difficulty in the clinical environment and with his wife at home. However, when he is in situations where he is talking with someone other than his wife, he becomes so fearful that he will not be able to comprehend what is being said to him that he cannot tolerate the situation. Further, his high level of anxiety in these situations interferes with his ability to use his strategies to increase his comprehension, thus reinforcing his belief that he can never function outside the home. The new behaviors to increase comprehension are not generalizing to other environments. Determine what problems you see in this situation and set forth a plan of action which will resolve the problems. Again, you will find a discussion of these situations in Appendix C.

Chapter 7

Synopsis

The CIM is not limited to individual therapy or individual interactions with a client. It also applies to group therapy. Group therapy takes many forms in our field and some forms are more effective and efficient than others. The *shaping group*, a unique and new form of group therapy, has been developed specifically to emphasize the advantages of group therapy and minimize the disadvantages. This chapter demonstrates the differences between types of group therapy and then demonstrates the strengths of the shaping group. Operational and procedural guidelines of the shaping group are presented so that you will be able to create such a group.

Chapter 7

Group Therapy

DEFINITION OF TERMS

Over the years that I have supervised therapy, I have seen many forms of what is referred to as "group therapy." This term is applied whenever a speech clinician is working with a group of clients. I have classified these various forms of group therapy into three rather distinct categories: "mob therapy, therapy in groups, and group therapy." Let us discuss each form of therapy so we can identify it when we see it.

When we discuss mob therapy, we will apply the OP Rule since we know that this applies only to the other people we have observed. In this type of therapy, the clients form a "mob," not a group. The mob runs the group and the therapist is controlled by the mob. The theme of this type of therapy is "chaos." No one, not even the clinician, knows where the mob is going or the purpose of getting together. The mob interaction is impossible to follow since there is no purpose. You can always tell when you are observing mob therapy because the clinician has a bewildered look on her face as she frantically attempts to control the mob. As the mob gets further out of control, the bewildered look of the clinician turns to panic and then to hysteria. Needless to say, this form of "group therapy" accomplishes nothing. Mob therapy is not all that rare among speech clinicians.

Therapy in a group is the most common form of "group therapy" practiced by the speech clinician, particularly in the public school environment. This is partially due to the role models of teachers and students found in this environment. The clients are expected to play a passive role in the classroom as the teacher assumes the more assertive role. When the children come for therapy in a group, they behave as they would in the classroom. They sit and wait for the speech clinician to organize the group activities, decide who will receive therapy in what order, and make the decision as to the correctness or incorrectness of speech behavior. In other words, the speech clinician is performing individual therapy *in* the group. The clinical process applies directly to this situation since we are still in an individual therapy mode. The reason that the children are brought to therapy in a group is for the efficient use of the speech clinician's time. It would be extremely inefficient for her to have to go to the classrooms and get each child individually.

Group therapy implies an interaction between the members of the group. It also implies that the members of the group are directly involved in the therapeutic process, both in terms of receiving therapy and providing therapy. This form of therapy evolved from the field of psychology where treatment is provided *by* the group. The group interaction focuses on the sharing of problems and possible solutions. This therapy form is rarely used by the speech clinician.

GROUP THERAPY FOR THE SPEECH CLINICIAN: THE SHAPING GROUP

A unique form of group therapy, the *shaping group*, has been developed during the past several years. We will discuss this group therapy process rather briefly in this book but there are two sources you can turn to for an in-depth review of the shaping group (Leith, 1979, 1982). First of all, let us contrast the shaping group with the more traditional form of therapy in a group (from now on referred to as a therapy group).

Contrasts in Group Treatment

Group member's activities. In a therapy group, the clinician is working with one client at a time. The other members of the group are, we hope, listening and watching the therapy. They are waiting for their turn to receive therapy. Supposedly, this listening and watching activity has some therapeutic value. However, Mowrer (1972) found that these listening and watching activities have no therapeutic value. The clinician provides the modeling, guidance, and information, makes all of the judgments as to the correctness of the individual's responses, and administers the reward or the penalty. There is little, if any, group interaction. If there is group interaction, it often means that the clinician has lost control and we are back to mob therapy. The only learning that takes place is when the individual members of the group receive their individual therapy from the clinician. The model for the therapy group is seen in Figure 11.

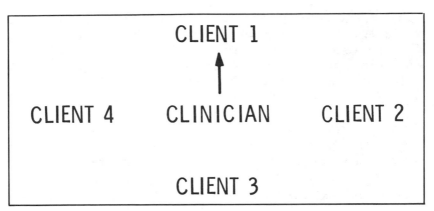

FIGURE 11
In-group treatment with the clinician providing individual therapy for Client 1. Clients 2, 3, and 4 are watching and listening. This type of clinical activity is of questionable value (Mowrer, 1971). (Reproduced with permission from Leith, 1979.)

In the shaping group, each member of the group is actively involved in the CIM. They are involved in providing the modeling, guidance, and information for each other. They also make judgments as to the correctness of the responses and apply either the reward or the penalty. There is constant interaction between the group members. In essence, each member of the shaping group is playing two roles: as a clinician when the group is focusing on another group member, and as a client when the group is focusing on them. In that the group members are constantly involved in the shaping group, learning is an ongoing process for all group members during the entire group meeting. Figure 12 illustrates the relationships in this form of group therapy.

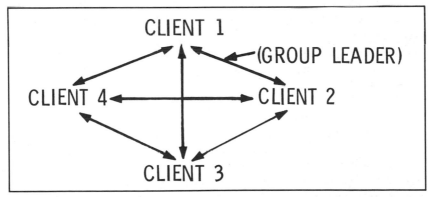

FIGURE 12
The Shaping Group configuration with the Group Leader monitoring group activity, directing group focus, modeling appropriate responses to behaviors, and performing other tasks of the Shaping Group Leader. Client activities consist of performing and monitoring new speech behaviors, rewarding or penalizing behaviors of other group members, participating in group discussions, and other forms of group interaction. (Reproduced with permission from Leith, 1979.)

Self-monitoring activities. In the therapy group, the clinician makes all of the judgments of the correctness of the member's behaviors. She addresses the issue of teaching listening skills on an individual basis, and the only time the group member engages in this new skill is when he is receiving his therapy.

Group members in the shaping group are constantly involved in using their listening skills. Not only are they monitoring their own speech production, they are applying their listening skill to the speech of all other group members. One of the objectives of the shaping group is to teach all group members to listen carefully and judge the correctness of speech production. Self-monitoring is an extremely important part of generalizing the new speech behavior to other environments. The shaping group carefully teaches this skill.

The clinician's tasks. In the therapy group the clinician's tasks resemble those which we discussed earlier in individual therapy. The clinician does most of the talking, unfortunately, often to the point that the client cannot get a word in. The treatment mode has not changed, we just have some other people listening to and watching the therapy.

The tasks of the clinician change drastically in the shaping group. She is no longer performing direct therapy on the members of the group. Rather, she is teaching the members of the group to function as clinicians through modeling, guidance, and information. The CIM applies here even though she is teaching behaviors other than speech behaviors. As the group members learn to function as "clinicians" in the group, the clinician assumes a more passive role, allowing the group to do therapy with a minimum of modeling, guidance, and information from her. She now spends most of her time monitoring the group interaction and providing assistance only when the group needs it. The most difficult part of this new role for many clinicians is to be quiet and not monopolize the group interaction. Have you ever thought about how much the clinician talks in a clinical session as opposed to the client? Who is supposed to be practicing their speech in these sessions?

Individual and/or group therapy. With a therapy group, the clinician has no choice between therapy modes. She is doing individual therapy at all times. With the shaping group the clinician has two distinct modes of therapy, individual therapy with a client or the shaping group process. The question that arises is when should she use the different modes. Let us turn back to our five steps in treatment: evaluation, determining the behavior change goal, getting the behavior to occur, habituating the behavior, and generalizing it. The first two steps are not involved in the clinical process so we now have to decide where to introduce the shaping group during the three final steps in treatment. It is probably more efficient to work individually with the client in getting the new behavior to occur and then begin the shaping group at the habituation stage. This does not mean that the new behavior cannot be taught in the group, but this tends to be a therapy group rather than group therapy. As long as the clinician is aware of this so that she can shift back to the shaping group after the behavior has been taught, there is no problem. This is discussed in greater detail when we address the issue of adding new members to the group.

Types of Shaping Groups

Due to the wide range of ages of our clients, and other factors, there are four rather distinct types of shaping groups. Each type has some unique features based primarily on the ages of the group members. The most convenient way to indicate three of the types of groups is to relate them to the school level where the group's members would be. Thus, we will discuss the *elementary shaping group*, the *junior shaping group*, the *senior shaping group*, and the *adult shaping group*.

Elementary shaping group. The elementary shaping group is for children between the ages of 5 and 11. Because of the lack of social maturity of children of this age, this group should not exceed three members. The range of ages in this group is also critical. If possible, there should be no more than a 3-year age range among the members; however, the maturity of the children will influence this range. The clinician should consider this factor when starting an elementary shaping group. The male/female ratio does not seem to be too important with this group, although it is an important factor in other group types.

Junior shaping group. The junior shaping group is made up of children between the ages of 12 and 15. At this age there is more social maturity and the group size can be increased to four members. This group can tolerate a 4-year range of ages of members. However, a factor that must be considered is that this is the age of puberty; and puberty has strange effects on otherwise perfectly normal children. So, the male/female ratio becomes very important in this age group. Only the clinician can determine how to mix such a group and she must take into consideration the clients' ages, their degree of social maturity, and how they relate to the opposite sex. The junior shaping group calls for some careful planning.

Senior shaping group. Clients between the ages of 16 and 19 are appropriate for the senior shaping group. We have to limit this group to four members, not because of puberty but because of a new factor called *peer pressure* and its effect on group interaction. In some instances, where the clinician has a mature group of clients, she may increase the size of the group to five. The range in ages of the group members is now a very important factor. Peer groups seem to frown on interactions with younger persons. So if a group consists of three 18-year-old clients and one 16-year-old client, there might well be a problem with group interaction. The age range depends on the makeup of the group and is controlled by the clinician. Sex also rears its ugly head again. The male/female ratio is very important and an equal distribution seems to be the best way to handle the situation. As with the junior shaping group, this type of group calls for some careful planning.

Adult shaping group. Clients from the age of 20 on fit into the adult shaping group. We have finally reached a level of social maturity where we can increase the size of the group to a maximum of six members. The only limitation we have here is the ability of the clinician to deal with increasingly complex group interactions. We are also no longer concerned about either the age range of the group members or the male/female ratio in the group. This is usually the most stable of all the types of shaping groups.

Mixing Types of Communicative Disorders

If we happen to be able to create a shaping group where all the members have the same communicative disorder, we find that there are some advantages. If all group members are stutterers, they have a common bond and, since they all understand how it feels to be a stutterer, there can be a close interaction. They can share feelings and attitudes since all members of the group "understand." If all group members have a problem with the [s] sound, it makes it simpler to provide modeling, guidance, and information since it applies to all group members. Grouping clients by type of disorder has some advantages, but also some disadvantages. For example, a group of children who stutter might be a very difficult group to get interacting. They would shy away from penalizing the incorrect speech behaviors in order to get the new speech behaviors to occur and would tend to be quite nonverbal.

Does this mean that mixing clients who have different problems lessens the efficiency and effectiveness of the shaping group? No. It simply means that if the members of a shaping group have different disorders, the clinician must train the group members to recognize different speech behaviors. This is all part of listening skill and is related to improving self-monitoring. A client with a voice disorder can certainly make a judgment about language structure and respond with a reward or a penalty. The process is a bit more complex but still operational.

Activities of Group Members

The clinical process cannot operate effectively in the group unless all group members participate in the group interaction. This means that they must monitor the speech behaviors of other group members in order to respond with either a reward or a penalty. This is a major change from the client's activity in a therapy group. The members not only must know what the behavior change goals are for all group members, they must know which behaviors are to be rewarded and which are to be penalized. This information is provided for the group members by the clinician as she identifies each group member and what behavior they are working on. This is accomplished during the initial stages of the organizations of the shaping group and is the basis for training the group members to listen to both *what* is said and *how* it is said; all of which forms the base of self-monitoring. As the self-monitoring skills improve, the members' speech performance in the group will also improve, since they will be better able to judge their speech performance.

In that the group members have not had experience in providing reward and penalty for others' speech behaviors, they will have to be trained to do this. They will learn this both through the information given to them by the clinician and through observing the clinician as she initially models the presentation of the rewards and/or penalties. The most difficult thing to teach here is the presentation of the penalty. It is not too difficult to reward someone for a good job, but it is difficult to penalize someone. This concept is best presented to the group members by explaining that they can help other group members by reminding them not to perform the incorrect behavior. This reminder is in the form of a penalty and, since no one wants to be penalized, they will remember not to perform the incorrect behavior.

The strength of the rewards and penalties is crucial to the shaping group and their strength is dependent upon the participation of all group members. In that the group members form a peer group, the rewards and penalties are very meaningful, much more so than a reward or penalty from the clinician. Because the group members are peers, there is strong approach motivation to achieve peer rewards and equally strong avoidance motivation to avoid peer penalty.

Finally, all group members must participate in group discussions. These discussions provide each group member with an opportunity to practice his new speech behavior in a conversational mode. Since the topic of group discussion will also change, members can use their new speech in talking about a variety of topics, some of which might well take on emotional overtones. This will afford the members with yet another dimension of speech on which to practice their new speech behaviors.

Activities of the Group Leader

Many of the activities of the group leader have already been alluded to in previous discussions. It is a new clinical role which makes different demands on the clinician. She is no longer the clinician in an individual therapy setting. She is now a guide, a moderator, a supervisor. In a previous article on the shaping group as related to the treatment of stuttering (Leith, 1979), 16 unique tasks of the group leader were set forth. In this chapter we discuss some of the more meaningful ones. It is already apparent that the clinician must carefully set forth the rules and guidelines for the operation of the shaping group. During this time she must also identify the speech behaviors and the behavior change goals for all group members. Once the group process begins she must also maintain a balance between rewards and penalties in the group interaction. This last task is important so that the clinician can maintain the approach motivation and avoidance motivation of the group members. As the shaping group progresses she must make sure that the criteria for rewards and penalties change so that shaping can occur through successive approximation. This will necessitate guidance of the group interaction, and furnishing additional information to the group members. Finally, the group leader must be able to allow the group to interact without her constant input. If the group is functioning well, they really do not need her input. The amount of involvement of the group leader in the group interaction will differ according to the age and maturity of the group members.

Operating the Shaping Group

Instructions. In order to avoid mob therapy it is necessary to provide some rules and regulations. The group members must be instructed about how the group will operate, particularly what they must do to be a member of the group. The most important thing that must be established is that all members must participate in the group interactions. This is also where the group leader introduces the concept of presenting rewards and penalties. A difficult concept to teach, but one that must be established, is that behavior change goals are achieved gradually. The group members must understand that the new speech behaviors introduced in the group will be learned in steps, not all at once. This is the concept of successive approximation.

Identification of behavior change goals. The group leader must present each group member individually, discuss carefully what the incorrect speech behavior is, how far the group member has progressed, and what the behavior change goal is. This is an essential part of starting the shaping group, since the clinical process is dependent on the application of rewards and penalties to the appropriate behaviors.

Rewards and penalties. The group must decide on what they will use as rewards and penalties before the group procedure can begin. The members must make "educated guesses" at what they would find rewarding and what would be penalizing. The group leader will be able to verify their guesses after the group process begins by observing the effects of the rewards and penalties on the behaviors. It is very important that the group members themselves decide (with some not-too-subtle guidance from the group leader) on the reward and the penalty, since they will be the recipients. The rewards and penalties must be easy to apply, not take too much time, and not interfere with the group interaction. The best thing might be some sort of auditory signal such as a hand clap for a reward and a finger snap for a penalty. Visual signals are difficult to use, since, if the recipient is not looking at the person administering the reward or penalty, they will not perceive it. It is very difficult to maintain constant eye contact with three or four people at the same time. Token economies work very well here, since the tokens meet the criteria mentioned above and the backup rewards are better able to meet the variety of rewards a group might well demonstrate.

Getting the group started. After all of the instructions are given, the group members' behaviors identified, and the reward and penalty determined, we are ready to begin the shaping group. Since we are at the habituation stage of therapy, each group member is able to perform the new speech behavior but is still very dependent on the reward. The clinician must make certain that the group begins with a strong reward orientation. She should start the group by introducing a neutral but interesting topic for discussion. She might then ask each group member to comment on the topic. At this early stage of the group she might have to provide some guidance to make sure that the new behaviors occur. And when they do, she models the presentation of a reward for the group members. As the discussion continues she not only continues to model the presentation of the reward for the new speech behavior, she also rewards group members who start to reward other group members. The presentation of a reward by a group member is a new behavior she wants to encourage. She does this by rewarding it when it occurs. When the group members begin to reward each other for their new speech behaviors, the group is off and running and the clinician can fade her modeling. The group members are now providing their own modeling. The clinician can then assume the role of group leader; monitoring, guiding, and so on.

If penalty is needed in the shaping group, it should not be introduced until the group is operating smoothly. As the group members become involved in the discussion topic they may forget to produce the new speech behavior. This is when the penalty should be introduced. Remember, we only penalize an incorrect behavior when we are certain that the client can produce the correct behavior.

Variations in Group Organization

As soon as the group is stable, the clinician should train various group members to act as group leader. This works even with the elementary shaping group. Give them a little power and they fit right into the leadership role. Once the clinician has a couple of members who can lead the group, there are several variations in the group organization which add to the versatility of the shaping group.

In order to train a group member, the clinician appoints a particular member to lead the group. She then provides guidance as the new group leader learns to lead the group. She gradually fades her role as group leader as she transfers the role to the new leader. This group member then provides a model of a group leader for the other members of the group. The process is repeated until the clinician has as many new group leaders as she feels she needs. She can now vary the group organization. This variation in group organization is shown in Figure 13.

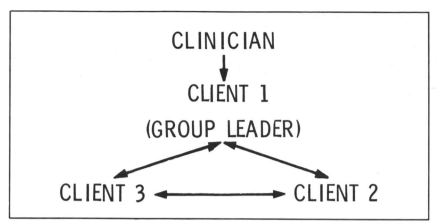

FIGURE 13
The Clinician is involved in training Client 1 to function as the Group Leader. The Clinician assists the Group Leader in maintaining Shaping Group interaction. (Reproduced with permission from Leith, 1979.)

If a member of the group needs some individual attention, the clinician can turn the group over to the new group leader while she provides the needed individual therapy. The group can proceed with therapy without the clinician being present. Of course, this procedure should not go on for extended periods of time but most clinicians who use the shaping group are amazed at how well the group can do without them. This form of the shaping group is shown in Figure 14.

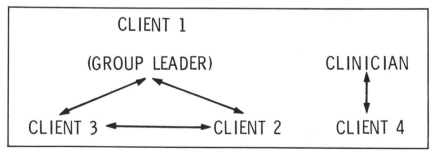

FIGURE 14
The Clinician is providing individual treatment for Client 4 while Client 1, acting as Group Leader, maintains the Shaping Group interaction. (Reproduced with permission from Leith, 1979.)

It is often wise for the clinician to sit back and observe the group interaction and the performance of each client. She can do this by allowing a member of the group to lead the group while she observes. In this way she can plot the progress of each group member, make changes in the group structure if necessary, and determine if the general direction of therapy is correct. This is illustrated in Figure 15.

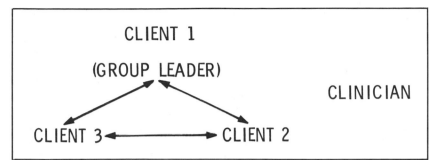

FIGURE 15
Client 1, acting as Group Leader, maintains the Shaping Group interaction while the Clinician observes and evaluates the group function. (Reproduced with permission from Leith, 1979.)

There is also the possibility that the clinician has too many clients to make up a shaping group. Let us imagine a group of six in an elementary shaping group. There are just too many children to make the shaping group work. So the clinician assigns three of the children to form a shaping group. She then assigns the remaining three children to serve as individual *monitors* of the three children in the shaping group. The monitors' job is to sit behind their "client" and monitor his speech. They are to remind him to use the new speech when he enters the group discussion. They are also to provide rewards and penalties to their "client." Although the monitors are not directly involved in the clinical process of the shaping group, they are learning listening skills, learning to monitor the speech of their "client." This will directly influence their ability to monitor their own speech.

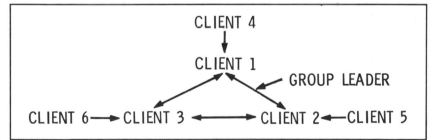

FIGURE 16
Clients 1, 2, and 3 are receiving a concentrated group shaping effort. They are receiving not only reward and penalty from group interaction but also constant feedback from their individual monitors, Clients 4, 5, and 6. The Group Leader performs routine tasks as Shaping Group Leader and also monitors the feedback among clients. (Reproduced with permission from Leith, 1979.)

After a period of time the clinician has the children reverse their roles, with the monitors becoming the shaping group, and the group members becoming the monitors. As shown in Figure 16, all six children are directly involved in therapy, not just listening to and watching the shaping group operate.

Adding New Members to a Group

Once a shaping group is in operation, it becomes an ongoing therapy procedure. Over a period of time, some members of the group will be dismissed from therapy. This does not mean that the group ceases to function. Rather, it means that we must add a client to an ongoing group. The new member has to be instructed as to how the group operates and who is working on what. This information is best presented by the remaining group members and can be accomplished in one clinical session. This is a good way to have the group members remind themselves of the purpose of the group and their responsibilities. The group then resumes therapy and the new member learns to function in the group through modeling and guidance from the other group members. The process is repeated each time a new member is introduced to the group.

The Clinical Process and the CIM

If you go back to the CIM you will find that it is operating within the shaping group, only in a more complex form. The stimulus, in the form of a question, may come from one group member. The member to whom the question was directed thinks about it and then responds. His response is then the stimulus for *all* of the group members and they evaluate it and respond. The strength of the reward or penalty is increased because it is being administered by a number of peers. However, the strength may vary from time to time. If we have a group of four clients, they may not all agree that a behavior was correct. In this event, only those who felt the behavior was correct would respond. We now have the possibility of a range of from one to three rewards being presented. Weaker rewards (one group member) indicate that the behavior is not as stable as it should be, while stronger rewards (three group members) indicate that the behavior is very stable.

As the speech behavior transactions continue between group members, the clinician also monitors the attending behaviors of the group members. She judges their approach motivation and avoidance motivation. If she finds a problem with either approach motivation or avoidance motivation, she can alter the rewards or penalties accordingly or focus the group on the attending behaviors of an errant group member.

It is important to note that all members of the group assume special stimulus roles. Through the presentations of rewards they become S+ and through penalties they become S-. The group members retain these stimulus roles when they leave the clinical environment. If members encounter each other in another environment, they cue each other so that the new behaviors are encouraged to occur, and the occurrence of the incorrect behaviors is discouraged. In this way, the shaping group provides valuable assistance during the generalization phase of the clinical process. This is of particular value in the school environment where the group members encounter each other during the school day. As you can see, the CIM extends beyond the clinical environment since all group members retain their stimulus roles outside therapy.

Chapter 8

Synopsis

There are many instances in our clinical contacts where our clients, or even their significant others, have attitudes, emotions, feelings, or other cognitive sets which interfere with our therapy. As professionals, we should not only be able to recognize when these factors are influencing our therapy, but we should also be able to deal with some of these factors without making a referral for counseling. It is just as important that we are able to recognize when we have reached our counseling limit and need to make a professional referral. However, we often find it difficult to make a professional referral because of lack of professional recognition by other professionals or their lack of interest. This chapter addresses these issues and offers some techniques and procedures to use when faced with these problems.

Chapter 8

Attitudes, Emotions, and Feelings

Earlier, I discussed the client's cognitive process and how it might possibly work against our therapy. In this discussion, I dealt with the client's attending behaviors, that is, what he was attending to in the clinical environment. If the client is not attending to us and our therapy, we cannot operate either effectively or efficiently. But there is another side to the client's thinking process which can also have a negative effect on our therapy. This has to do with the *cognitive set* of the client. The cognitive set represents the client's attitudes about himself—his emotional reactions to himself and his environment, and his emotional reactions to the interactions between these factors. This obviously does not apply to all of our clients, but if a client's cognitive set is negative, this could influence our therapy, both in form and substance.

If we go back to the "dead man" rule to define a behavior, then thoughts are behaviors. In the behavioral literature they are referred to as *coverant* behaviors. This word is a contraction of the words *covert* and *operant*. So we will use the term coverant to mean behaviors performed by the client which we cannot observe. We are talking specifically about the client's thoughts, his cognitions. And the particular cognitions we are concerned with here are those which form the client's cognitive set; his emotions, attitudes, feelings, fears, self-concept, and self-confidence. For the cognitive set that is essentially negative in nature we will use the term *negative coverants* (negative thoughts) in our discussion.

A natural question for the speech clinician to ask is, "Do we work with negative coverants in our therapy?" Let me break this into two questions. First, are we confronted with negative coverants in therapy and, second, do we work with them? Let us consider the first question concerning the presence of negative coverants in therapy. With many of our clients there are no negative coverants which we must consider in planning our therapy. But even with these clients, they can appear abruptly and have a devastating effect on therapy.

Consider the 7-year-old client with an articulation disorder who has been a joy to work with in therapy. Might there be a change in the client if the parents were suddenly divorced? Could this situation have an influence on the client's self-concept, self-confidence, and security? And could these negative coverants adversely affect therapy? The answer is "yes." Maybe we can do nothing to change this child's negative coverants, but we should be aware of their influence on our therapy.

With some clients, but definitely not all of them, the negative coverants must be an integral part of therapy. Our therapy must deal not only with the speech behavior but also the "emotional problems" of the client. May I use the term emotional problems without having you conjure up images of severely emotionally disturbed people? At this point in our discussion I want to talk about our clients who have emotional problems but are not disturbed to the point where they need psychological or psychiatric treatment. We will get to the disturbed type of client later in our discussion. What type of client might have negative coverants severe enough that they would cause emotional problems? This could be the client who has had a laryngectomy, the client who has had a CVA, the client who stutters, or the client with cerebral palsy. The list could be expanded to include any client who has negative coverants related to his disorder which interferes with therapy.

How do negative coverants interfere with therapy? There is an endless list but some of the more obvious ways are by distracting the client from therapy tasks, negating the client's motivation, creating deep states of depression or anxiety, and undermining self-confidence. We cannot ignore these negative coverants if we are concerned about the efficiency and effectiveness of our therapy. We must include, as part of our treatment program, the modifying of the negative coverants to the point where they no longer interfere with our treatment of the communicative disorder.

MINIMIZING NEGATIVE COVERANT INFLUENCES

Behavioral Intervention

Since coverants are learned behaviors, as are operant behaviors, they can be modified the same way. That is, the contingent event (reward or penalty) will influence the frequency of occurrence of the coverant. The problem is that coverant behaviors cannot be directly observed. Let us illustrate this concept for the sake of clarity. We will consider the speech clinician who has just parked her car in her agency's parking lot. She is just getting out of the car when a man, parking behind her, bumps her car so hard that the tail light is broken. Does she become angry? Yes. I forgot to tell you that she does not own the car. It is her boy friend's brand new car and he is a fanatic about keeping it neat and clean. Now, the question is, how does the other driver know she is angry? Anger is an emotion and a coverant. The emotion is manifested in operants that are observable. The operants reflect the coverant. Our speech clinician gets red in the face, she increases the loudness of her voice (that is, she is yelling), she restricts her vocabulary to shorter words (most of the four-letter variety), she stamps her foot, pounds her hands on the car, and displays other operant behaviors that reflect her anger. So operant behaviors can reflect coverant behaviors. This principle can be used to modify the negative coverants of our clients.

As our clients talk to us about their attitudes, feelings, and emotions, they will be overtly expressing their cognitive set, their inner thoughts. If we then reward or penalize certain thoughts, they will increase or decrease in frequency. Of course, we must be very careful of the type of penalty we use in this situation, since the client might interpret the penalty as being directed to talking about a negative thought, and the result would be that the client would just not talk about it. The following is an example of a conversation with an adult stutterer where the principles of reward and penalty are used to modify the client's negative coverants. You will be able to follow the interaction if you consider it as a series of transactions. We will be following the CIM. The only difference is that the client's response is the expression of an attitude, feeling, or emotion rather than the production of a specific speech behavior.

Counseling Session with Stutterer

Clinician: How is it going with using the new speech when saying your name?

Stutterer: I am afraid to try it. If I stutter, the listener will think I am retarded or stupid.

Clinician: You mean that some people think stutterers are retarded or stupid?

Stutterer: Yes, most people think that way.

Clinician: I don't agree with that. Most people just don't understand what the stutterer is doing and they do not know how to react.

Stutterer: You really believe that people do not view stutterers as retarded or stupid?

Clinician: Yes, I do. And research in listener attitudes shows that only a very few listeners feel that stutterers are retarded, stupid, or something of that nature.

Stutterer: I sound and look stupid when I stutter.

Clinician: I have seen you stutter many times and I do not see you as being stupid.

Stutterer: I am not stupid, I am very intelligent.

Clinician: Yes, I agree. I think you are very intelligent. You have understood all of the concepts I have taught you. You catch on very fast.

Stutterer: But, this is why I get angry when people think I am stupid. I can tell what they are thinking when I watch them.

Clinician: No, you cannot tell what they are thinking. You can only guess. And I think your guesses are wrong. You see a strange look on someone's face when you stutter to them and you guess that they think you are stupid. Maybe, their expression is only because they were surprised when you stuttered.

Stutterer: Maybe I am guessing at what they are thinking. I really do not know what they are thinking for sure.

Clinician: Right! No one is a mind reader. And since you are so sensitive about your stuttering, you might just read things into your guess that are just not there. Could you try and be a bit more fair to your listener and give him or her the benefit of the doubt?

Stutterer: I can try but it will be very difficult. What I could do is see if I could read other things into people's facial expressions. Maybe I said something funny and that would be the reason for the expression, not that they think I am stupid.

Clinician: I think that is a great idea! You might see if you think the person is embarrassed because they do not know how to react to you, or if you caught them by surprise, or if they are just very curious since they have never seen a person stutter before.

In the above interaction you find the clinician rewarding the more positive coverants of the stutterer and penalizing the negative coverants. This same approach could be used with the aphasic as he makes statements to the effect that he can never be of any use to society again, that he is a burden to everyone, that he is helpless, that he will never get any better, and other such negative coverants. It can also be used with the client who has had a laryngectomy and is in a deep state of depression about his future. The clinician's rewards and penalties are used to modify the client's cognitive set and to increase approach motivation and avoidance motivation in the client.

There is a great deal of cognitive input from the clinician in this type of interchange. Going back to the CIM, the clinician provides the client with modeling, guidance, and information. The same principles and concepts in the CIM apply as we modify the client's cognitive set. There are a number of methods of cognitive intervention that the clinician can use.

Cognitive Intervention

Modeling/guidance. When we provide a model of a behavior we are dependent on the client perceiving it on a cognitive level. He must perceive it in such a way that he is able to associate it with his own behavior and then imitate the model. This is a valuable way of dealing with fears associated with certain types of stimuli. Let us talk about fear associated with snakes. Most people have a negative reaction to snakes. We are not born with the fear of snakes; we learn it from a variety of sources. One way to overcome the fear of snakes is to observe a person handling snakes who has no fear of them. The person provides us with a model of how to pick up a snake and handle it. Then, if we can work up enough courage to try it, we find that by imitating the person we gain confidence and lose fear of handling snakes. If we are working with a stutterer who has a great fear of the telephone we can model the correct way of answering the telephone. Our client "attacks" the telephone when he is answering it. He grabs it and is trying to say "hello" as he is bringing the receiver to his ear. Most stutterers are sensitive to time pressure, being rushed to respond, and here we see the stutterer putting himself under time pressure by rushing to answer the telephone. We break the act of answering the telephone into several different steps and remove the time pressure. We model the act by first looking at the telephone, putting our hand on the receiver, picking it up, placing it to our ear, and then saying "hello." We model this so that the client can see how to perform the act correctly.

As the client imitates the model, we provide guidance to help him. We use verbal, gestural, physical, and environmental guidance to assist the client in his attempt to imitate our model. We want him to succeed and this prompting will increase his chances of achieving success.

Information. We used behavioral information as part of the strategy in the modification of speech behaviors. Now we can use general information to present the client with information to change a negative coverant. For example, this can be used to great advantage with the client who is going to have a laryngectomy. There is a great apprehension about what life will be like after surgery. The speech clinician should discuss this with the client before surgery to reassure him that he will be able to communicate after the laryngectomy. There is a great deal of information available that the clinician can present to the client in order to set his mind at ease. Negative coverants can exist with almost any disorder. The professional literature provides all of the information we need to counsel our clients. We simply must recognize our responsibility to deal with these issues.

Talking it out. When we have a client who is not "emotionally disturbed" but who has "emotional problems" that he wants to talk about, do we automatically refer him to a psychologist or psychiatrist? No. First of all, we should talk with the client. There is nothing better than to have someone to talk to about things that are bothering you. The entire world is looking for a good listener. I will make this a more personal message. Let your clients talk to you about their problems. Use your special talent, your common sense, and you will recognize when the client's problems are such that you should make a professional referral. But, for the most part, just being a good listener will help the clients resolve some of their problems. One common source for talking out problems for the general public seems to be the bartender at the local bar. All he does is listen and nod his head. How can you go wrong if all you do is nod your head?

Using your common sense, you can also discuss the client's problem with him. How many times have you sat down with a friend and helped him/her work out an emotional problem? You listened, offered opinions, analyzed what your friend has said, or presented alternatives. You served as a sounding board. Why can you not do this with most of your clients who have problems? There is no reason except that we have the mistaken feeling that we are stepping out of our professional limits. We only step out of our professional limits when we attempt to delve into problems beyond our capabilities or when we ignore the emotional lives of our clients. I am not suggesting that we play the role of psychologist or psychiatrist. I am saying that we must be aware of our client's cognitive set and sensitive to the presence of emotional problems. We can deal with them to the best of our ability in therapy or refer those clients who need professional help to a psychologist or psychiatrist.

I counsel my clients in terms of their emotional problems. I have also referred clients to professional counselors. But I will deal with the problems first to see if I can resolve them or modify them within my clinical setting, since once the client is referred to another professional, it is very difficult to coordinate the two treatment programs. I attempt to deal with my clients' fears, self-concepts, self-confidence, attitudes, and feelings. I let them do the talking and respond as I suggested you do with friends. I consider myself a speech clinician who works with clients who have communicative disorders. Therefore, I must work with both the client and the disorder.

There are some *technicians* in our field who work on only the communicative disorder and ignore the client and his needs. Unfortunately, these technicians often hide under the guise of performing behavior therapy; but once you remove the humanistic element from therapy, you end up being a technician. These people can be replaced with a machine that dispenses rewards. Therapy is based on a human interaction which includes attitudes, emotions, and feelings.

As long as we approach our clients with a positive and helpful attitude, we are not going to create additional problems by talking with them about their current problems—no more here than if we talk with our friends about their problems. Who knows the most about the various types of communicative disorders and how people feel when they have the disorder? The speech clinician. How effective will the psychologist or psychiatrist be in working with an aphasic, a stutterer, or a person with a laryngectomy when he does not really understand the disorder or the emotions related to it? Give yourself credit for your professional training and standards, and deal with your client's cognitive sets.

Inventory: Assets and liabilities. One of the best ways to objectify something is to write it down. If you are feeling "down in the dumps," get out a piece of paper and write down what is bothering you. You will be amazed at how quickly you can change your attitude once you examine the things that are bothering you. Things will not appear as foreboding once they are written out. We can use this same technique with a client who has a negative cognitive set toward himself. I have my clients write out a detailed list of assets and liabilities.

I tell them not to rush this, to take their time in getting the list to me. The longer they take, the shorter the list of liabilities (but they then include procrastination as a liability). When the list is finally turned in, I go over it with the client and we talk about each item to see how valid it is. I often find that stuttering clients take a characteristic such as "sensitivity" and put it in the column of liabilities. They insist that they are too sensitive to other's reactions. I do not argue the point but I point out that sensitivity to other's needs and feelings can be viewed as an asset.

Group sharing. If you are in the position of providing group therapy for your clients, you have an opportunity to work on your clients' emotional problems by allowing them to share their problems. Whereas one client might have a problem in one area of his life, he might have some insights into problem areas of other clients. Group discussions of a particular client's problem provide the client with insights as to how others have dealt with the problem. The clinician will need to monitor the group discussion and clarify points or point out possible difficulties with suggested solutions. However, if the group members are all active in discussing each other's cognitive sets, all members of the group profit from the experience. If the group is homogeneous, with all members having the same communicative disorder, the discussions are much more to the point and meaningful since they are all sharing a common problem. This type of group is especially good with stutterers, aphasics, and laryngectomees. I have found it advantageous at times to have the group comprised of clients who are just entering therapy as well as clients who are well advanced in therapy. The more advanced clients can provide valuable insights for the beginning clients. Then there is the issue of credibility. The client is more apt to listen to another person who has resolved a similar problem than to the clinician who has never experienced the problem.

Referrals for Professional Counseling

To supplement speech therapy. Yes, Virginia, there is a psychologist—or a psychiatrist—and she can help us when we are experiencing difficulty with a client. We will be faced with clients whose emotional problems are such that we cannot deal with them, but they are interfering with therapy. So we decide to make a referral for counseling as we continue with our therapy. This decision and procedure will most often be dictated by the agency where we are employed. The family is also involved in the decision making. Who do we refer the client to? This question may also be answered for us by the agency. If you find yourself in such a situation and have a choice in terms of the referral, I have some suggestions. The most important criterion in this instance is to find a psychologist or psychiatrist who will work *with* you. You must coordinate your therapy with the counseling the client is receiving. This calls for good communication between you and the counselor. This is not always easy. I have found it wise to have a meeting with the psychologist or psychiatrist to discuss coordinating the two treatment programs. One sure sign of a bad choice for a referral is that the individual will not take the time to have a conference with you. I have also found it very important that the psychologist or psychiatrist appreciate the role of my profession and respect me as a professional. If I do not get this, I know I will not be able to coordinate the treatment programs.

When you decide that you want to refer a client for counseling, consider the orientation of the person to whom you might refer your client. You will find, generally, two basic orientations for treatment. One is psychodynamic, which means that the treatment is based on a personal interaction between the professional and the client. There is an exchange of concepts and ideas which, through guidance by the professional, leads the client to a resolution of the problem. The second orientation is psychoanalytic, based on Freudian concepts. The more typical analytic approach is very nondirective. The analyst responds to the client by nodding or by encouraging the client to continue talking. The two treatment methods are vastly different. You may wish to seek some consultation on this matter before you make your referral.

The other choice you have is between a psychologist and a psychiatrist. The psychologist is not medically oriented and cannot prescribe medication. She has majored in psychology for many years and has either a masters or doctorate degree. Her orientation is almost always psychodynamic.

The psychiatrist is a physician who has specialized in psychiatry. She is an MD who can prescribe medication and often includes this as part of her treatment. The psychiatrist may have either a psychodynamic or a psychoanalytical orientation. Let me point out that a person becomes an analyst only by going through many years of analysis themselves. This is not an academic program. The psychiatrist receives the MD degree with a specialty in psychiatry through a university training program which is academically oriented. To become an analyst, the psychiatrist must undergo several years of analysis from an analyst. Only upon completion of the analysis can the psychiatrist advocate her treatment as psychoanalysis.

In place of speech therapy. There are also situations where you decide that the client needs professional counseling before he is ready for speech therapy. With this type of client there are so many emotional problems in the client's life that he cannot effectively deal with your treatment. You may attempt to work with the client but your therapy is not producing the desired effects. The client behaves in bizarre ways and most of your therapy is out of your control. I have seen speech therapy like this, but where the client has no emotional problems. We discussed this earlier as "awful" therapy performed by other people.

If you find yourself in a situation like this where the client's emotional problems prevent your working with him, this is the time to make a referral. It is not as important here to find a professional who will communicate with you, since you are not attempting to coordinate two treatment programs. But it is wise to make sure that there is some communication so you know when you should reintroduce your treatment program. Again, this must be coordinated through your agency and the family. Your actions depend on the policy of the agency where you work.

DEALING WITH UNPROFESSIONAL PROFESSIONALS

We have only dealt with the emotional problems of the client thus far in this chapter, but we must consider our own problems before we conclude our discussion. I am not talking about the general run-of-the-mill problems such as uncooperative clients, or the client's significant others, or the working conditions, or equipment that does not work, or other clinicians who do not work. I am talking about the frustrations we have when we attempt to deal with other professional workers who not only do not understand our profession and the services we provide, but are not interested in learning about them. We encounter this problem working in environments where we work in conjunction with other professions such as teachers, physicians, occupational therapists, physical therapists, psychologists, nurses, and counselors. These people provide us with valuable supportive services and they have a significant influence on the motivation of our clients. If they are supportive of us and our therapy in their contacts with the client, they provide valuable assistance by helping the client maintain his motivation. But if they are either directly or indirectly critical of us and the services we are offering the client, we have a problem of maintaining the client's motivation. These are *our* significant others in the professional environment. We need the support system that they form within this environment, but how do we accomplish this? My experience has been that the professional people who do not support my clinical efforts do so not because they are malicious, but because they do not understand our profession. We are faced with an educational task, one where we provide special information to the other professionals with whom we work. We might view this as *public relations* within the professional community. If we put on a good public relations campaign, we can expect nothing but positive results. This does not mean that we cram our information down the throats of the other professionals. We do not *confront* other professionals with their lack of understanding of our profession. Rather, we make information available in the most acceptable and professional manner. For the professional who is receptive to learning about other professions, this will suffice. However, we will not be able to educate all of the professionals with this approach. There are those who will never be interested in anything but their own area and there is no way to educate them. Ignorance is Bliss. Think of how many blissful unprofessional professionals you have come into contact with. These are the ones who frustrate us. Following are some ways we can attempt to educate these "uneducated" people.

One of the best ways I have found is the agency in-service training program. Most of the professional staff attends these training programs. What better vehicle do we have than having these people as our "students"? But make sure you are well prepared for the program. The professional staff you are trying to educate probably comes with a negative bias and if you are not prepared and do not do a professional job, you only confirm their original negative feelings.

Another approach which I have used is a person-to-person discussion of a clinical problem with various staff members. When they are asked for their advice on a problem, they are flattered and become interested and involved. You do not have to follow their advice, just ask for it. Who knows, you may actually get some excellent advice and you will both have learned something. This is a good opening for a discussion where you can provide them with information they do not have and have not requested.

Letters and reports are another good avenue for us to provide information to other professionals. This means that the letters and reports must be well written and manifest high professional standards. A poorly written letter or report does more damage than good. If this is your only means of communication with other professionals, write carefully and clearly, eliminate as much professional jargon as possible, and edit your work before the final letter or report is submitted.

Finally, I would suggest that we are on a two-way professional street. If we are asking other professionals to understand what our profession is all about, we should also understand what the other professions are about. It is embarrassing to find a speech clinician who is working in a rehabilitation agency who does not understand the difference between occupational and physical therapy even though she works with both professions. If we are asking others to be more professional, we should require this of ourselves. "People who live in glass houses should not throw stones."

DEALING WITH PROBLEMATIC SIGNIFICANT OTHERS

Significant others sometimes tend to interfere with therapy with their negative attitudes and responses to the client's particular communication disorder. In previous chapters we have discussed shifting their role from an S– to an S+ or an S0 by changing their response from a penalty to a reward or at least a neutral response. In most cases the negative response on the part of the significant others is not meant to be disruptive, it is a response that comes naturally from frustration, from not understanding the nature of the client's problem. We can assist the significant others most effectively by providing them with information about the client's disorder. We can also tell them how to respond. For example, the parents of a young stutterer may respond to the client's stuttering by becoming frustrated and angry since they do not understand that the client cannot say the word properly. They constantly yell at the client to "stop stuttering." When the parents understand the nature of stuttering and that the client really wants to say the word but cannot, they will more than likely be able to change their response. We could even tell them to be patient with the client and give him time to get the words out. Significant others are not out to destroy your therapy, they are just human.

However, there are some significant others who may purposely work against your therapy because of their own needs. They may be so emotionally involved with the client and his disorder that they respond rather irrationally. I was once working with a 6-year-old severely involved cerebral palsied girl and part of my treatment consisted of teaching her to feed herself. I would make very good progress during each therapy session but when the child returned for the next session, she had lost everything I had taught her 2 days earlier. This went on for about 2 weeks when the social worker in the agency called me in for a conference on the child. She had been working with the mother on her emotional involvement with the child. The mother had a great deal of guilt associated with giving birth to a severely handicapped child. She compensated for her guilt by waiting on the child constantly. She would even get up every hour during the night and turn the child over. The child became her "crown of thorns," her source of punishment for what she had done.

As the child became more independent and did not need her help as much, the mother felt she was losing her "crown of thorns," which she needed in order to deal with her guilt. One of the things she was doing in order to maintain the child's dependence on her was to slap her hands if she attempted to feed herself. I then understood why I could not achieve progress with the child. The mother had established herself as an S– for self-feeding behaviors. Obviously, this situation could not be corrected by giving the mother information about the disorder. The mother needed professional help in dealing with her emotional problems associated with her handicapped child.

Although this type of situation may be the exception rather than the rule, these clinical situations do exist and must be dealt with in a most professional manner. If you do not have a social worker or a psychologist in your agency to turn to, you might contact the family physician and seek his advice. Just be certain that you operate within the rules of the agency where you are working. In this type of situation, the significant other needs as much help as the client.

Finally, there are those significant others who are undermining your therapy due to some personal factor unknown to you. You find that you are making no progress because of the responses of the significant others and you have no way to change their attitudes or responses. They reject even the most subtle reference to counseling. What do you do here? This depends again on your agency. If you have a waiting list of clients who would profit from your therapy, you must consider how to make the most effective and efficient use of your clinical time. You may have to dismiss the client, as regrettable as this may be, so that another client can profit from therapy. I once worked with a young stutterer and was making very significant progress when the father suddenly removed him from therapy. I discussed this with the father, but his only response was that his child would just have learn to live with it and "be a man." He justified his yelling at the child by explaining that it "toughened him up." No amount of discussion would change the father's attitude. This is a situation you must just accept, regardless of the moral and ethical issues involved. Child abuse takes many forms.

References and Recommended Readings

Bandura, A. *Principles of behavior modification*. New York: Holt, Rinehart & Winston, 1969.

Beck, A. T. *Cognitive therapy and the emotional disorders*. New York: International University Press, 1976.

Bloomer, H. Professional training in speech correction and clinical audiology. *Journal of Speech and Hearing Disorders*, 1956, *21*, 1, 5–11.

De Cecco, J. P. *The psychology of learning and instruction: Educational psychology*. Englewood Cliffs, NJ: Prentice–Hall, 1968.

Fitts, P. M. Factors in complex skill learning. In R. Glass (Ed.), *Training research and education*. Pittsburgh: University of Pittsburgh Press, 1962.

Gazda, G. M. (Ed.) *Basic approaches to group psychotherapy and group counseling*. Springfield, IL: Thomas, 1970.

Gentry, W. D. (Ed.) *Applied behavior modification*. St. Louis: Mosby, 1975.

Hill, W. F. *Learning: A survey of psychological interpretations* (3rd ed.). Scranton, PA: Chandler, 1971.

Holland, J. G., & Skinner, B. F. *The analysis of behavior: A program for self-instruction*. New York: McGraw–Hill, 1961.

Kazdin, A. E. *Behavior modification in applied settings*. (Rev. Ed.). Homewood, IL: Dorsey, 1980.

Lazarus, A. A. *Behavior therapy and beyond*. New York: McGraw–Hill, 1970.

Lefrancois, G. R. *Psychological theories of human learning: Kongor's report*. Monterey, CA: Brooks/Cole, 1972.

Leith, W. R. The shaping group: Habituating new behaviors in the stutterer. In N. J. Lass (Ed.), *Speech and language: Advances in basic research and practice* (Vol. 2). New York: Academic Press, 1979.

Leith, W. R. The shaping group: A group therapy procedure for the speech/language pathologist. *Communicative Disorders*, 1982, 7, 8, 103–115.

Levis, D. J. *Learning approaches to therapeutic behavior change*. Chicago: Aldine, 1970.

Martin, G., & Pear, J. *Behavior modification: What it is and how to do it.* Englewood Cliffs, NJ: Prentice-Hall, 1983.

Meichenbaum, D. H. *Cognitive behavior modification: An integrative approach.* New York: Plenum, 1977.

Mowrer, D. E. Accountability and speech therapy in the public schools. *Asha,* 1972, *14,* 111–115.

Norman, D. S. *Memory and attention.* New York: Wiley, 1969.

Parker, C. A. *Psychological consultation: Helping teachers meet special needs.* Leadership training institute/Special education, University of Minnesota, 1975.

Perkins, W. H. (Ed.) *Current therapy of communication disorders: General principles of therapy.* New York: Thieme/Stratton, 1982.

Staats, A. W., & Staats, C. K. *Complex human behavior.* New York: Holt, Rinehart & Winston, 1963.

Vargas, J. S. *Behavioral psychology for teachers.* New York: Harper & Row, 1977.

Parker, C. A. *Psychological consultation: Helping teachers meet special needs.* MN: Leadership training institute/Special education, University of Minnesota, 1975.

Appendix A

LEITH'S LAWS OF THERAPY

1. The probability that your therapy will be observed by a supervisor is directly related to your lack of preparation for therapy.

   COROLLARY: Your best therapy sessions are never observed by a supervisor.

   COROLLARY: Clients cancel or fail to appear for those therapy sessions you are best prepared for.

   COROLLARY: The number of toys and games taken into a therapy session by a clinician is inversely related to her degree of preparation for therapy.

2. When a child becomes ill in therapy the probability that he will throw up on you is directly related to how recently you had your clothes cleaned.

3. Children are the most hyperactive and difficult to control in therapy on those days you are not feeling well.

   COROLLARY: Children who you first judge will be pleasant to work with prove to be the most difficult clients you have.

4. When your therapy is planned around a piece of equipment, it will be missing or not operating on the day you need it.

   COROLLARY: When you need a piece of clinical equipment for therapy, it will be checked out by the clinician just before you.

5. Your best ideas for therapy occur just after you have finished writing your therapy plan.

6. The last client of the day always is the one who needs the most clinical time.

7. The more difficult it is for you to get to work due to the weather, the more likely your clients will fail to appear for therapy.

   COROLLARY: Your client who misses the most appointments will keep his appointment on the day that you are absent because of illness.

8. Errors in client reports will not be noticed until the report is through its final typing.

9. When a clinical secretary is replaced, all files and final reports are lost for a period of no less than two months.
   POSTULATE: Clinical files disappear in direct relation to their importance.

10. Your absent client will arrive for therapy immediately after you have poured yourself a cup of coffee.
    COROLLARY: When you go to get a cup of coffee during your only break in therapy for the day, the person just before you will have emptied the coffee pot.

11. You become a professional speech clinician only when the time you spend on paper work is equal to the time you spend in therapy.

12. When a piece of a test is misplaced, it remains lost forever.
    COROLLARY: Tests only lose their validity when more than 50% of the test is missing.

13. Lights are turned on behind one-way mirrors only when the client is looking into the mirror.
    COROLLARY: The time you decide to rearrange your clothes in the clinic room is that time when there are several observers behind the one-way mirror.

14. After all desirable rooms in an agency have been assigned, the speech clinician has the choice of all remaining space.
    COROLLARY: Speech clinical rooms must be located next to a bathroom, an elevator, a gymnasium, or a band rehearsal room.

15. Clinical equipment sent out for repairs never returns.

16. Power cords used to connect clinical equipment to wall outlets disappear after three months.
    POSTULATE: Power cords that disappear are impossible to replace since no one manufactures a cord that matches the equipment.

17. If a piece of equipment operates on batteries, the batteries are always "dead" when you need to use the equipment.

18. When writing a diagnostic report from your notes, the data you most need will be on the piece of paper you threw away when you finished the evaluation.

19. The one cassette tape that jams in your recorder and is destroyed will contain your most important clinical recording.

20. By the time you become aware of your client's wiggling and squirming in his chair it is most often too late.
    COROLLARY: The previous law applies 10-fold when you are holding the young client on your lap.

21. When school assignments are made for itinerant school speech clinicians, the older the clinician's car, the further apart the schools will be.
    COROLLARY: School assignments for itinerant clinicians are based on the longest possible drive from the clinician's home.

22. The day you wear a skirt to work will be the day your clients will require you to work on the floor with them.
    COROLLARY: On that day you have worn a skirt and are working on the floor with your clients, you will have observers, most of whom are male.

23. When carrying your clinical materials to or from a clinic room, the item you drop will be the most fragile and the most expensive.

24. When you are late for a clinical appointment, your client will arrive twice as early as you are late.

25. When chocolate is used as a reward in therapy, clinicians give themselves more rewards than they give their clients.

26. Electrical outlets in clinic rooms are always located at the farthest point from the work table.
    COROLLARY: Power cords for tape recorders and audiometers are always six inches too short to reach the wall outlet plug.
    COROLLARY: All electrical extension cords disappear the day you need them.

27. The theories and therapies we were taught never apply to the clients we are working with.
    COROLLARY: Our specific clinical problems are never discussed in any journal or reference book.

NOTE: There will be periodic new editions of Leith's Laws of Therapy. You are invited to contribute to future editions by sending your suggestions to Dr. William R. Leith, Communication Disorders and Sciences, 573 Manoogian Hall, Wayne State University, Detroit, MI 48202.

Appendix B

LEITH'S WMEOANRINDGSS

1. TEETH   TEETH

2. PIT
     CH

3. MUCOUS
   CLEFT

4. **TONGUE**

5. NASAL L
          E
          A
          K

6. (LIP, LIP) "AH"

7. NODE
   CORDS

8. MANNERISMS, *mannerisms*

9. PECTORALIS
   pectoralis

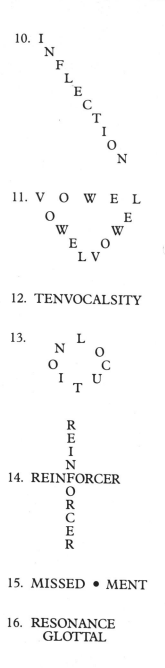

10. I
      N
       F
        L
         E
          C
           T
            I
             O
              N

11. V   O   W   E   L
       O   E
        W   W
         E   O
          L V

12. TENVOCALSITY

13.   L
        N   O
       O   C
        I   U
          T

          R
          E
          I
          N
14. REINFORCER
          O
          R
          C
          E
          R

15. MISSED • MENT

16. RESONANCE
       GLOTTAL

17. SEYRNRTOARX

18. WORD + FINDING =

19. NORMAL WITH LIMITS

20.
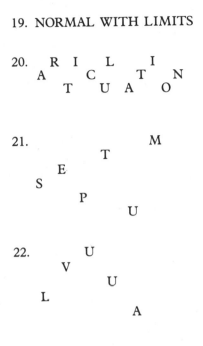

21.

22.

NOTE: The answers to the word games in Chapter 2 are as follows:
1. Cleft palate
2. Up in pitch
3. Multiple artic errors

The answers to the WMEOANRINDGSS above are given below. They are upside down so you cannot cheat and look ahead. You will also find out the hidden meaning of WMEOANRINDGSS in this section.

Answers to WMEOANRINDGSS: (1) space between the teeth, (2) pitch break, (3) submucous cleft, (4) macroglossia, (5) post-nasal drip, (6) bi-labial sound, (7) node on the cords, (8) secondary mannerisms, (9) pectoralis major and minor, (10) falling inflection, (11) vowel triangle, (12) vocal intensity, (13) circumlocution, (14) positive reinforcer, (15) missed appointment, (16) supra glottal resonance, (17) error in syntax, (18) word finding problem, (19) within normal limits, (20) distorted articulation, (21) deviated septum, (22) bifid uvula. You must look for the hidden meanings in words.

Appendix C

PLANNING AND DISCUSSING PROBLEM SOLVING

There are no standard answers to the following situations. What follows are my interpretations of the clinical problems and how I might approach them. You may indeed have a better approach than I. This section is meant as an exchange of ideas, so compare my "answers" with yours and try to determine why there are differences.

Chapter 4

Situation A. The 17-year-old male presents several problems as we attempt to determine what an appropriate stimulus will be. Our first consideration must be the influence of the possible hearing loss on his perception of the sound in the words we are trying to teach him. Our clinical goal is to teach him a basic vocabulary that others in his environment can understand. If his hearing loss is so severe that our model of a word is extremely distorted, he may produce the word in such a fashion that it still cannot be understood by others. This would be the first test. We may also find that the hearing loss is not a significant influence. We might get some distortion but the listener can still identify the word.

If there is too much distortion in the auditory channel, we might supplement this input with physical guidance of the oral structures in the production of the word. We may even have to break the words down into the individual sounds and teach them through a combination of modeling and physical guidance.

We do not have any information about the cognitive function of this client, but we would be suspicious since there is a history of brain injury. Both the modeling and physical guidance call for cognitions on the part of the client. If the modeling and physical guidance fail to produce the correct response, we might then add some verbal guidance, giving the client some hints about how he might change his speech attempt to make it correct. As a last resort we might add behavioral information, but this is at a rather high cognitive level.

With this client we want to avoid as much as possible our dependency on the auditory channel and high cognitive function. These are the two factors which are most suspect. Therefore, we turn to stimuli which are more visually or physically oriented.

Situation B. Our 45-year-old laryngectomized client poses some very interesting problems. First of all, how are we going to teach esophageal speech? We can provide behavioral information to the client but this is all very abstract. How can you verbalize production of this form of speech? It would be better if we provided a model at first so the client can see and hear what we are doing in order to produce the "voice." After the client has seen and heard the model, the behavioral information is much more meaningful. This is why it is so very important that the speech clinician be able to perform all of the special behaviors she is asking her client to perform. Without the model, the learning process is going to be very slow and frustrating. We are already dealing with a client who is depressed and he does not need any additional frustration. We can supplement the model and the behavioral information with verbal and physical guidance as the client attempts to produce esophageal speech. Still, the most important stimulus is the model of esophageal speech.

Our client is depressed and this has a negative influence on our therapy. We can use both general and behavioral information to attempt to offset the depression. We provide the client with information about others who have had a similar operation who have then gone on with a successful career. We give the client positive statistics and facts about the disorder. We can also approach the depression by using our contingent events. There is nothing better to ward off depression than success. And success is even sweeter when there is a meaningful reward associated with it. We must plan our therapy carefully so that the client is successful. He must see that he is able to succeed in modifying the disability, and then he must receive a meaningful reward.

Situation C. What do we do with a 7-year-old who has everything? We will find it very difficult to work with approach motivation to achieve something. We are probably going to have to turn to avoidance motivation with this child. We are going to have to find something she wants to avoid and then cultivate her avoidance motivation. Our contingencies are going to be penalty oriented and her reward will be to avoid the penalty, a negative reward. For example, let us say that the child enjoys playing a certain game with us in therapy. We tell the child that we will play this game at the end of each therapy session but she will have to "buy" the game so we can play. We then give her 10 tokens and say, "Here is some special kind of money we will use to 'buy' the game. You have 10 tokens and the game costs 7 tokens. You can 'buy' the game with the tokens you have. But we have to learn a new sound first and if you are not paying attention to me I will take a token away from you. If you do not have 7 tokens at the end of our speech work, you cannot 'buy' the game and we will not be able to play." This is "response cost," where her nonattending responses cost her a token.

Now, there is also the chance that we could use the game for approach motivation if she really wants to play it. In this event we would reward her for attending to therapy. She would be told that she would have to have a certain number of tokens in order to "buy" the game so we could play. We would then give her tokens for attending to therapy. This token economy is reward oriented while the previous one is penalty oriented.

There is also the possibility that we can combine both rewards and penalties. In this token economy we would reward the attending behavior and penalize the nonattending behavior. This might be the best approach we could use since we would be both encouraging attending behaviors (approach motivation) and discouraging nonattending behaviors (avoidance motivation).

Situation D. In order to teach this 9-year-old boy to produce easy vocal onset (easy vocal attack) we should provide him with a model. This means that as a clinician we must be able to perform this behavior. We select a single vowel sound and produce it with a hard and an easy vocal onset so the client can hear the difference in production. We then would ask him to attempt to imitate the easy vocal onset. If his attempt is close to the model we may be able to shape it by providing him with some guidance, primarily verbal and gestural. We might tell him to make the transition into the vowel slower, and indicate this by a hand gesture. We could also repeat the model, slowing down the behavior so he can hear how we gradually introduce vocalization.

What would we do if we could not produce the behavior ourselves? We would have to depend on behavioral information. We would explain carefully how to produce easy vocal onset. This could be accomplished by telling him to start with an [h] sound and then move into the vowel. If we had selected the [eɪ] vowel, we would tell him to say the word "hay" very slowly. The next step would be to gradually reduce the duration of the [h] sound until, for all practical purposes, it no longer exists and the [eɪ] vowel is produced with easy vocal onset. During the course of shaping the easy vocal onset we would also use guidance, both verbal and gestural. The only thing missing here is our model of easy vocal onset. However, we could use this same technique to train ourselves to produce the easy vocal onset behavior. There really is no reason why we cannot provide a model of this behavior. Speech clinician, heal thyself.

Before we close this case, let us consider what other things we would do to reduce the amount of vocal abuse that is occurring. If we decided that we also wanted to alter the habitual pitch, we would again use modeling, guidance, and information as we changed the pitch of the voice. In terms of other forms of abuse such as too much yelling and shouting, we would rely primarily on information about how this injures the vocal folds. In other words, we would give the client a lecture on vocal hygiene and hope that this would have an impact on his use of the voice. We attempt to influence this client's attitudes and beliefs regarding the use of his voice. This is basically a form of counseling and it takes the form of changing the client's cognitive set about how he views his voice. There is an exchange of attitudes and beliefs between us. We must first of all determine how he views his voice before we can attempt to change his views. This is only one of many clinical experiences where we have to work on the client's cognitive set as well as on speech behaviors.

Chapter 5

Situation A. The removal of the prompt from this 50-year-old client should not pose any serious problems. We gradually remove the stimulus or prompt. If we suddenly remove the prompt, the word may indeed fail to occur, so we remove it in gradual stages. Let us suppose that the gestural guidance prompt is to pretend to drink water from a glass. The prompt consists of our pretending to pick up a glass, lift it to our mouth, and then tilt it up so we can drink from it. We can gradually remove the prompt by eliminating the final step, the tilting of the glass. We can even gradually remove the last step by not tilting the glass as far, or not moving our head back as far. We remove the prompt in steps small enough that the client can maintain the response as the prompt is removed. We shorten the duration of the stimulus by making each successive prompt less complete. With some clients we may be able to remove the prompt in large steps, while with other clients we have to create very small steps.

Situation B. Our problem with the 13-year-old client with cerebral palsy is that we moved too fast when we went from a continuous reward to a 2:1 ratio. We suddenly reduced the presentation of the reward to 50% of occurrences of behavior. It would be much better if we changed the ratio of reward more slowly. Our first step might be to go to a 10:9 ratio, rewarding 9 occurrences and then passing over the 10th performance. When the behavior is maintained with this ratio we can reduce it to 10:8, then 10:7, and so forth. After we have reached the 1:1 ratio we can shift to a 2:1 ratio where he is rewarded for every other production. This can continue through 3:1, 4:1 ratios, and so forth, until the reward is eliminated and the behavior continues to occur.

Situation C. The 15-year-old male who is going through voice change is reacting to peer pressure and we must help him through this difficulty. We should deal with it while he is still in the clinical environment so we can control the variables in the speaking situations. Role playing can be used with this client. We can start by having him use his new pitch while pretending to talk to a person who is not threatening to him. We can play the role of the other person. We can then work our way up through more intimidating people. This might be followed by having another client come into the clinical room to talk with the client. Then we might bring in a couple of clients. We gradually introduce those talking situations where the client is afraid to, or cannot, produce the new pitch. As the client is successful with the talking situations in the clinical environment, he will experience less tension and more confidence in those talking situations in the external environment. The gradual presentation of these talking situations helps the client generalize the behavior to environments outside the clinic room.

Chapter 6

Situation A. There are a couple of problems we face in attempting to generalize the new speech of our 67-year-old laryngectomy client. He is depressed about the effects his speech will have in his social contacts and, since he is a widower, he has no support system to help him generalize his speech to other environments. First of all, we should have dealt with the social impact of his speech earlier in therapy. We will have to deal with this by giving him general information about others with his condition. We might even arrange to have someone who has had a laryngectomy visit the client and talk about how he has adjusted. The introduction to another person with the same condition does wonders for morale.

The other problem we face is the lack of a support system. With no wife in the picture, we could ask about his close friends. He may have some friends with whom he meets with on a regular basis. Perhaps they meet daily to play cards or some other activity. We might ask our client if he would bring a close friend with him to therapy. We could then formally, or informally, create an S+ for our client by shifting the stimulus role of the friend. The formal creation of an S+ could only be done if the client agrees to it. We would explain that his friend could help him remember to use the new speech, and he could also tell the client how well he was speaking. Again, we must remember that our client can use esophageal speech, but only in the clinic room. If we can introduce some of our client's friends into the treatment program, we can create a support system and get the new speech to occur in other environments.

Situation B. Our 14-year-old female is not only dealing with a voice disorder; she is dealing with puberty, a new female role, and peer pressure. Fortunately, she has a support system in that her parents are concerned and willing to help. She is caught in something of a "trap" situation. If she uses her old voice, people laugh or tease her about it. At the same time, if she uses her new voice, she is often teased because the voice is so different. All of this is going on during those sensitive, early teenage years. One would think that the new voice would be so pleasing that she would use it immediately in other environments; but there are ambivalent emotional factors that pull her in two directions.

Since we have the cooperation of her parents, we should start introducing the new voice in a highly controlled environment, the home. We will shift the roles of the parents to that of an S+ by having them give her verbal praise when the new voice occurs. We should be able to establish the new voice in this environment without too much trouble since we have the cooperation of the parents. Our next step would be to have our client bring a friend home and use the new voice with her friend in this structured environment. We could then increase the number of friends brought into the home, controlling the sex makeup of the group. If our client feels more comfortable with female friends, we might start increasing the number of females in the group. Males could be introduced either as members of the group of friends or as a single male friend brought to the house. As we gradually introduce the new voice into our client's environment, she will not experience the tension which prevents her from producing the voice in outside situations.

Situation C. Our approach to this 58-year-old male with a receptive language problem would be quite similar to the one we used with our 14-year-old voice client. We must gradually introduce other talking situations in order to allow the client to gain confidence. We are fortunate in this instance, since the new behavior is occurring in the home environment. We strengthen this circumstance by making our client's wife a very strong S+ through a heavy reward program.

We then gradually modify the home environment by bringing in other people. We might start with a close friend and carefully control the content of the conversation so as to prevent it from getting too abstract. The topics of conversation would then be varied in order to increase the demands on comprehension. The number of friends brought into the house would then be gradually increased and the topics of conversation controlled as before.

As our client is gaining confidence in the home we would instruct our client's wife to take him along on her various shopping trips and while doing errands. We would instruct our client to enter into small conversations with people in these different environments. In that the wife is with him and is a strong S+, she will cue appropriate behaviors to occur and will provide much needed moral support for our client. She will also be able to intervene if a conversation begins to become threatening to our client. We are again introducing threatening situations in a controlled fashion, making certain that our client can succeed and gain confidence in these situations.

Index